Hot, Sexy and Safer

IS FOR EVERYONE . . .

. . . and here's what everyone is saying about Suzi Landolphi and her electrifying one-woman show that inspired this book!

"Your energy, enthusiasm, and knowledge of the subject are incredibly impressive . . . **Hot, Sexy and Safer** has given [us] a better understanding of safer sex, AIDS prevention, and sex education."
> —DAVE EMMONS, *Director of Student Activities,*
> *Southwest Missouri State University*

"Suzi was definitely a breath of fresh air that was desperately needed on this campus in terms of sexual awareness."
> —JOSEPH A. ORAVECZ, JR.,
> *Assistant Director Student Activities,*
> *Central Michigan University*

"Suzi Landolphi's **Hot, Sexy and Safer** . . . is educating thousands of adolescents about a very urgent and timely issue—safer sex."
> —*Center for Population Options,*
> *Washington, D.C.*

"You have made an impact on our campus. In a world turned topsy-turvy by this epidemic, your voice of sanity is valued."
> —W. JOSEPH JOINER, *MBA Director,*
> *Eastern Kentucky University*

"Holy mackerel!! What a show!! Suzi was fabulous! Through her performance, she really touched the students, entertaining and educating the entire time."
> —MICHAEL MINJARES, *New Student Programs,*
> *San Diego State University*

(continued)

"Suzi is the most unique one-woman show to have graced our community. Her approach to AIDS/HIV and STD education is absolutely moving. Three months after her appearance, I still hear comments from the participants on how great and useful her program was . . ."
—BOB AXELTON, *President, ASK, Inc.,*
Anniston, AL

"The five-hundred-plus students who came to see your performance seemed inspired . . . You gave such a positive message about their own and others' sexuality."
—CATHY CHARLTON, *Rutgers University*

"Watching Suzi seduce a group of ultrasophisticated medical students into understanding basic aspects of their own sexuality shows how she brings both light and heat to education. Reading her material reinforces her down-to-earth logic and commonsense understanding of anatomy, physiology and psychology and explains her straightforward appeal to her audience."
—NORMAN AMES POSNER, M.D.,
Director of Undergraduate Education,
Albany Medical College

"I would highly recommend Suzi and her program to any university or organization looking for a program that will address the intellectual, emotional, social, physical, and spiritual well-being of their students or members."
—BRIAN ASH, *Program Assistant,*
Sacred Heart University

Hot, Sexy and Safer

Suzi Landolphi

A PERIGEE BOOK

A Perigee Book
Published by The Berkley Publishing Group
200 Madison Avenue
New York, NY 10016

Book design by Irving Perkins Associates

Cover design by Pamela Tauss

Cover and interior photographs by Caroline Greyshock

First Perigee edition: September 1994

Published simultaneously in Canada.

Library of Congress Cataloging-in-Publication Data

Landolphi, Suzi.
    Hot, sexy, and safer / by Suzi Landolphi.—1st Perigee ed.
      p.   cm.
    "A Perigee book."
    ISBN 0-399-51882-7
    1. Safe sex in AIDS prevention.   I. Title.
  RC607.A26L355   1994
  613.9—dc20   94-11087
                                 CIP

Printed in the United States of America

10 9 8 7 6 5 4 3 2 1

Mom,

I wrote a book! I hope you can read it from your heavenly view. There's so much of you in here: your wisdom, love of life, respect for one's self and others, your delightful sense of humor, and your belief in our ability as human beings to never give up on improving ourselves physically, emotionally, intellectually and spiritually.

As a little girl and young woman, I watched you struggle, fight and overcome every moment of despair with grace, courage and gentle, yet determined spirit. I miss you so much and could use your warm hug and encouraging words as I still struggle with my fears and insecurities.

In life, you were my mentor, a living example of the greatness which human beings can achieve. In death, you are my inspiration to not just try, but *do*. I promise you I will keep getting better, to become someone your granddaughter can emulate, and to carry on your tradition of caring for ourselves and others who share this universal struggle for love and the mysterious joy called life.

Your loving daughter,
Suzi

Contents

Acknowledgments   ix

Introduction: How I Became Hot,
Sexy and Safer Suzi   1

1. A Message from the Secretary of Sex   5

2. Free Your Mind and the Rest Will Follow   9

3. How We View Our Private Parts   17

4. Sex: The Wrong Way   29

5. Me and My Genitals   35

6. Learning to Masturbate, Again!   41

7. My Life with Erections   45

8. Intercourse Can Get in the Way of Great Sex   55

9. Sexually Transmitted Diseases   69

10. Safer Sex Is Better Sex   76

11. Condomania   89

12. They Make Sex Look So Easy on Television   108

13. Getting Real on Daytime TV   113

14. Orgasm Stress   119

15. My First Orgasm   124

16. Gay, Straight, Bi, and Other?   128

17. The Best Turn-on: Honesty and Trust   135

18. Sexually Act Your Age and Enjoy It   142

19. You Rub Me the Right Way   146

20. There's No Such Thing as a Silly
    Sex Question   152

    Two Very Personal Thank-Yous   161

Acknowledgments

I'm going to try to send out more thank-you notes. I carry around so many thank-yous that are never expressed to those I owe gratitude and appreciation.

Tina Mabry, my friend and business partner, always sends out thank-you notes and makes her kids send them out, too! She's right. Actually, Tina is right about most things because she believes in doing the right things for the right reasons. She also makes most things right. Like my life, for one. She has made my life better through the most successful means available to human beings—just living right. Tina lives with a balance of heart, mind and spirit. This is right. She does what she says she will do. This is right. She's honest. This is right. She is kind and generous. This is right. She believes in the best of us all and somehow gets it from all she touches. This is so right. Most everything that is right about Hot, Sexy and Safer—the performance and the book—has been co-created by Tina.

Now Tina will be embarrassed while she's typing these words, because she is also a very humble person. So, before you read this book, I need to let you know that, if you like it and it helps you on any level, and if you decide to write to me, or you see me on the street, don't forget to thank Tina, too. Thank you, Tina, for being someone I will always look up to and for being a friend who lives what is right.

Of course, there are others who have helped me too, so

here's my Hot, Sexy and Safer thank-you list to all those talented and special people.

To Lyle Gregory and Linda Shusett, you saw the value in Hot, Sexy and Safer before most others and have been champions of the most important issues of our times. You are guardian angels of this earth. For all those who don't know all that you do, thank you.

To Jim Pinkston, you believed in the Hot, Sexy and Safer message and brought it to the attention of the literary world. You made this happen.

To Jeremy Tarcher and his staff, you "got it" and helped me build my confidence as a writer and set me in the right direction.

To Mary Ellen Strout, you took my sometimes nonsensical words and sentence structure and added the wisdom of a strong and vibrant editor, woman and mother. Your insight provoked me to dig deeper and push harder.

To Daniel Nussbaum, you are a man who, on our first meeting, humbled me with your own personal triumphs and then dazzled me and my work with your outrageous wit and honesty. (To the Reader: write to the publisher and ask when Daniel will be offered a big book deal.)

To Donna Gould, your energy and enthusiasm makes me look and sound depressed! The world needs a million of you!

To Julie Merberg, I will never forget what you shared with me in your office, and every time I think about it, I have this big shit-eating grin on my face. You validated me and all women that day! From a white-paged, typed manuscript, you brought this book into the hands of every reader.

Gratefully acknowledged for their support of Hot, Sexy and Safer and me:

Stephen Michaels, condom king and friend.

Richard Bencivengo, never a playboy; a husband, father and friend.

John Walker, a man that every boy needs as a big brother.

John, Josie and Paul Politano, a true family that values all kinds of families.

My brother, Jimi, and Teri, for never doubting me.

My sister, Judy, Alex, Malcolm, and Brent, for being my family.

My dad, Charles Manuel, for loving my mother and being "Grampy" to my daughter and a real father to me.

GLAD (Gay and Lesbian Advocates and Defenders) of Boston and Neila Straub, you will make the words "and justice for all" become more than words.

To all the high schools, colleges and universities who had the courage to bring me to your campuses.

To Harry Collings, Liz Page, Gail Beverly and Jack Jerdan, you nurtured the idea of Hot, Sexy and Safer before it was a reality and stuck up for me and my work.

To Susan Kilmartin, no one draws better private parts than you! Thanks for your beautiful artistic touch every time we need one.

Many thanks to our friends at SIECUS (Sex Information Education Council of the U.S.), the Alan Guttmacher Institute, Advocates for Youth (formerly The Center for Population Options), the Division of STD-HIV Prevention of the Centers for Disease Control, Stephen Michaels Sales, and Okamoto USA for assisting us in gathering statistics.

Introduction: How I Became Hot, Sexy and Safer Suzi

• I'm in the car on the way to my performance, which starts in twenty minutes, and I realize I need condoms for the show. I ask the driver to pull over, and I run into the corner drugstore—*the* corner drugstore in Waterville, Maine. I'm in a really big hurry. I enter like a blast of winter wind and scan the store in two seconds. No condom rack! From a center aisle, I can see a little old lady behind the counter at the far end of the store.

"Excuse me!" My voice bounces off the old plaster walls and high ceiling. "Do you have any condoms?" She turns white. I can see the fluorescent light reflecting off her skin as the color drains from her face and neck. I'd better go to the counter.

"Do you have any condoms?" She nods, I think. Behind her fluffy hair, I see a few boxes. "I'll take all you have. Don't bother to put them in a bag, and I need a receipt. They're for my work."

• When you go through an airport security X-ray machine, condoms look just like . . . condoms! I carry about fifty or seventy-five in my shoulder bag. I love the shocked expressions on the faces of the people checking the monitor as my bag passes through the X-ray.

• I try to explain to the hotel clerk what I do. My credit card says Hot, Sexy and Safer. Thank God I have lots of luggage.

How It Began

Like many of the best things in life, Hot, Sexy and Safer started by accident. In 1983 I volunteered for an AIDS organization in Boston. Early in the AIDS epidemic, no one really knew what to do, except that people needed help. I was trained as a "Buddy." We cared for people with AIDS, comforting them when they felt sick, walking their dogs, mailing letters, doing dishes, being there when we could. After two years of Buddy work I was asked to be an AIDS educator. At the end of two weekends of intense training, I was ready to go out when an organization called for a speaker.

The trainer said, "Do it any way that you like, make it your own speech and your own style. Say it in your own words, and present the information in a way that's comfortable for you." I took him literally. I adopted an up-front, no bullshit, in-your-face style. I'd tell it like it really is, and when I thought it was appropriate and effective, I'd throw in some humor and wiseass remarks. I went to high schools a lot. I already knew about teenagers. My daughter and her friends filled my house like locusts eating everything in sight. I knew that when I got to the sex part of the speech, the kids were going to get nervous and embarrassed.

No one can stand up in front of 1,500 high school students and talk about anal intercourse, or any intercourse, and not make jokes. But using humor, I could deliver a message of sexual sanity and keep the level of embarrassment way down. A few parents got upset. Some people prefer ignorance. Some people want myth over truth. Sex is the only arena where intelligent people believe that we're better off *not* knowing the truth about a significant and complicated human expression.

Sex Jungle

Hot, Sexy and Safer grew, and soon it graduated and went to college. In five years I've visited over four hundred campuses and spoken live to over a million people. Now I'm so busy traveling the country talking about safer sex that I'm too tired to have any. The performance is an hour-and-a-half journey through today's sexual jungle. If it has anything to do with sex, I have something to say about it: how attitudes shape sexual behavior, how gender roles get programmed, what the big deal is about sexual orientation, what kind of sex is appropriate for young teenagers, why people will risk death to get laid. I talk about what we learn and don't learn from mass media, parents, school, friends, religion, and our own experiences. I cover a lot of ground, but I always wish we could explore more. There's never enough time. We can only hang out for so long. Besides, I want my audiences to leave feeling inspired, not as if they just heard a reading of the *Encyclopedia of Sexual Psychology and Physiology*.

Now I have enough time to say what I've always wanted to say: Hot, Sexy and Safer is a book. I've never written a book before. As a matter of fact, I've never even written down the text of my performance. It's very different for me to communicate this way. My audience doesn't have to leave after ninety minutes. And it's a lot quieter! No noisy crowd. No laughter. No smiles for me to see. No one blowing up condoms and batting them around the theater! It's hard doing this by myself, but I do get to share more. More of myself, more about things we rarely talk about, more about the things that scare us, hurt us, embarrass us, and keep us sexually stuck—stuck in ignorance, judgment, and guilt. More important, I can focus on how to get unstuck so we can create a sex life we are proud of, one that expresses love and caring and brings pleasure to us and our partners.

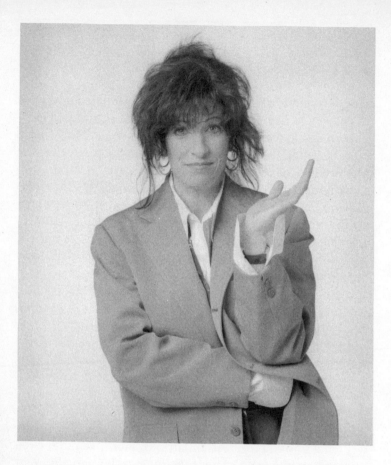

I never heard a woman say that she's worried she'll never find a big enough penis.

1

A Message from the Secretary of Sex

If Congress and the president created a new cabinet department and appointed me the Secretary of Sex, I already know what I'd do as my first official act. I'd send out a pamphlet to every home with the message: "Guys! Wake up! Nobody cares how big your dick is!"

Please. Enough wiener worry. I've never heard a woman say she's concerned that she'll never find a big enough penis. The biggest car doesn't necessarily give the smoothest ride. Let's put less emphasis on equipment and more on how you use it. Size doesn't have anything to do with how well you give or receive sexual satisfaction. Besides, unless you run into Lorena Bobbitt, you're stuck with your dick the way it is.

Happily, women's bodies can adapt equally well to penises of all dimensions. When a woman gets sexually aroused by having her clitoris rubbed, her vagina will react, too. First, it starts to quiver. Subtly, though; her whole body won't shake. The vagina will start to expand slightly, stretching and lengthening upward.

Now, let's say that a woman is getting close to having

an orgasm (because the clitoris is being stimulated), and let's just say that there happens to be a penis in there—or something like a penis! (At this point, the vagina really doesn't care if it's real or not.)

Walls Close In

As a woman gets closer to her orgasm, the clitoris gets bigger and harder, just like a tiny penis. Blood rushes into the walls of the vagina, which start to close in and get shorter again. Amazingly, the vagina will not stop closing in until it wraps itself tightly around the penis inside, whatever the size. So while you guys are worrying about Ralphie's size, our vaginas are busy taking up the slack!

A woman needs to feel truly aroused for this great system to work properly. Too many of us have intercourse *before* we, or our vaginas, are ready. Before clitoral stimulation. Before we know where our orgasms are. Before we have *all* the information about how we work. Before we are sexually proud and confident people. Before we have a true sense of our own self-worth. Before we understand that our physical, emotional, intellectual, and spiritual well-being is more important than our partner's orgasm.

A lot of people, male and female, simply don't know their bodies well enough to say what feels good to them. A man who can easily bring himself to orgasm may not know much about the possibilities of his own sexual satisfaction. Just because he can put his thing in her thang doesn't mean that he knows anything at all about women's sexual pleasure. Every man and woman needs to explore his or her body to discover individual centers of pleasurable sensation: the entire genital area, nipples, and other far-flung spots from head to toe.

Penis or Ramrod?

A lot of men treat their penises as ramrods, not ever discovering all the subtle nuances of touch and pleasure. A lot of women allow a penis in their vaginas way before they're physically, emotionally, intellectually, or spiritually ready. Vaginal intercourse is the easiest sexual act to do badly and a very difficult sexual act to perform well.

We need to do more sexual homework. Make that sexual home *play*. Home play should be fun. Finding out more about your sexual self can only lead to more sex information, more sexual self-confidence, and more sexual satisfaction, with no risk (other than having someone walk in on you at a most private time). In fact, knowing how you work, being able to give yourself an orgasm, and knowing where your best sensation spots are, will make it easier to show someone else how you work.

A Letter from All Women to All Men

Dear Friend:

Don't tell me that your orgasm is more important than mine, or that just because I can hold your semen in my vagina, I *have* to. It's not my lot in life to serve you sexually. I'm not responsible for your satisfaction; your hand can do the job, and so can anything else you choose to rub it with or put it into. Putting your penis in my vagina *may* do absolutely nothing for me sexually, and it *might* be putting my whole body, mind, and soul in a very bad place. Besides, my orgasm isn't in my vagina; it's on the outside of my body, in my clitoris. So don't lay "vaginal guilt" on me ("Oh, baby, you have to fix this!"), or give me "vaginal compliments" ("Baby, you feel sooo good"). They don't work, either. I'll let you know when, where, and how *I* want you to use *my* vagina. I'll be in charge of my parts, and you stay in charge of yours.

Don't use my vagina for an ego boost, stress relief, or a workout. My vagina isn't a place to retreat to when you feel pissed off at life. My vagina isn't a club whose membership ensures your place in the male race. (Yes, women use your penises for ego boosts too, and that's just as lame.)

Meanwhile, if we are going to get together, let's start by exploring all of our parts and places, because I just discovered a few more on myself that feel great. I promise to let you know when I'm getting turned on, and I want you to do the same. I promise to show you where my orgasm is and how I get it to work. I want enough light on to see your face and all your other parts. I want to move step by step, making sure that we don't skip anything and we don't move on until we get that particular sexual experience right for both of us. I know we can play to the point of orgasm without putting ourselves in danger of an STD or AIDS.

And if *we* decide to have intercourse, *we* will use a condom correctly. I've been practicing without you, putting it on everything in my house. Maybe we'll put a condom on you first and play with your penis before we put it in me! We can put some water-based lubricant, just a dab, on the inside of the condom before we roll it down, and it will feel so much better on your penis. I personally have grown to like the look of a condom on a penis, because I can feel freer—safer to let myself go. But don't forget to check it between thrusts, in case I can't see it from where I am, and I'll check it with my hands, too. As we tell each other how close we are to our orgasms, I'll remind you to pull out before you come, in case the condom breaks! By the time we do decide to have intercourse, I'll know when you're about to come, because I'll know and feel all your signs, but tell me anyway. And let's keep our eyes open, even during our orgasms. If you think we're ready to have intercourse, we should be able to look each other in the eyes.

With love and respect,
Suzi

2

*F*ree Your Mind and the Rest Will Follow

Once, as I was spouting off about this new sexual attitude stuff, a talk show host told me that my goals were "unrealistic." *Unrealistic?* What a cop-out. Talk about a bad attitude! When changes look or feel difficult, they're labeled unrealistic. Make goals seem unattainable and then we won't feel guilty for not trying to reach them.

We can choose to change our thoughts, attitudes, and behavior, any of which brings changes to our reality. None of us live in the same "reality" we did a year ago, five years ago, or ten years ago. As we gain new information, more experience, deeper insight, and sharper intuition, our reality changes. In fact, it's more realistic to expect our reality to change than to assume it won't. I've changed my reality more times than my hairstyle. And I know this for sure: a new sexual attitude is long overdue.

I've discovered in my work that learning about sex is a valid, authentic sexual experience. Okay, then. Let's have a real sexual experience—a Safer Sexual Experience, and a better sexual experience. *Safer sex is better sex!* And I can prove it. In fact, I wrote this book to prove it.

Let's Talk About Hot

Hot.   Describes something that has or gives off heat. But in Hot, Sexy and Safer, the word means much more. The most obvious meaning is sexual excitement, which also means being excited *about* sex. Hot—to have "an intense and immediate interest." A fresh approach, a new idea is *hot*! We're hot to *know* more about sex, not only to *have* more.

What's *Hot* and What's *Not*?

Hot	*Not*
Sexual self-confidence	Faking orgasms
Being in charge of your own orgasm	Being, or feeling, sexually used
Being proud of your private parts, i.e., gender positive	Hating your sexual orientation
Telling the truth	Telling lies
Condom stores	Sexually transmitted diseases
Self-satisfaction	Doing it with a partner in the dark under the covers with your eyes closed
Having sex information way before you start to "do it"	Homophobia, sexism, sexual harrassment, rape

Remember the childhood game in which someone hides something, and while the other person looks for it, the "hider" gives clues by saying "warm, cool, hot, or cold"? Well, Hot, Sexy and Safer reminds me of that game. Society and all of its institutions have hidden really important information about human sexuality—all the good stuff, like how we work, where our orgasms are, how to be sexually proud and confident, even how to be honest about sex!

Then, as kids growing up (as early as babyhood), we try to find it, and all society keeps saying is, "cool; cold; warm; no, cool again; very cold; *frigid!*"

"You Were Too Young"

Even when we get older and we're close to finding the stuff we need, we're still not getting very clear directions. No wonder we can't find it. And if by accident, years and years later, we stumble upon this great and important sexual information, what do the "hiders" say? "Oh, we figured you'd find it eventually. We were trying to protect and help you. We didn't want you to find it too soon. You were too young to understand."

Give me a break! We weren't too young to get pregnant or contract a sexually transmitted disease.

Hot means getting sex information before you use it. Our national habit of hiding detailed, clear, and honest sexual information keeps each generation ignorant. I intend to help break that national habit.

Just What Is Sexy?

Sexy.   A word loaded with meanings. My dictionary says: "*Adjective.* Sexually suggestive or stimulating; generally attractive or interesting; appealing." I wanna know who decides what gets labeled as attractive, appealing, or sexually stimulating. The advertising and entertainment worlds work pretty hard to pawn off *their* definition of sexy on the rest of us. I know that I, for one, don't meet all of their stringent criteria for the sexy woman. Height: tall enough to look down on most people. Weight: as low as possible. Perfect face, hair, skin, nails, voice, body movements, clothes, and look (as in come-hither-and-I'll-bring-you-to-ecstasy). And, lest I forget, breasts must be round and firm.

If you don't have 'em, go buy 'em. No cellulite (bumpy fat which, by the way, is a very normal female manifestation) on our butts. Few of us live up to these standards, so we believe we're "unsexy."

The Male Bimbo

Until recently, standards for male sexiness haven't been as strict. But then, if your gender is in control of most of the media, you can create unreachable standards for the other sex while setting lower standards for your own. History notes that most groups in power, be it a gender, a race, or a religion, have abused privilege at one time or another. But we live in a new era. Health clubs have filled with men who have learned the equation: crummy deltoids = death. Men, more than ever, are on display, parading across the stage in "up the butt" underwear. Commercials and music videos have created a new creature for the nineties; the male bimbo. Watch out, guys: living up to fake standards can make you cuckoo. Women learn quickly—and erroneously—that sexy is not how we feel, but how we look. Avoid the trap while you can.

Looks deceive. People who look very sexy might not *be* very sexy in terms of being comfortable with their own sexuality or anyone else's. And don't let their looks fool you or make you feel inadequate. I used to work on commercials, and I know that the models are styled, airbrushed, pasted, touched, retouched, and double retouched. I know that even the most glamorous ads are created by advertising agencies and paid for by manufacturers who care almost exclusively about selling more stuff. This is not a true sexy concept. Media images of toned, nearly naked women surrounding men who drink the right beer should not form our views about sex.

Remember—it's all make-believe. We can be sexy even if we're a little chubby around the middle and we drink tap water. What if the people who create these ads and the TV programs, films and music videos don't fit these idealized sexy standards either? Is that fair? Maybe we'd be less likely to compare ourselves to media sex icons that make us feel inadequate.

Back to the dictionary. "Sexy: Appealing. Stimulating." Works for me! This *sexy* is not about how a person looks. It's about new sexual ideas and information and attitudes. Appealing new attitudes about safer sex. A new kind of sex that can be *more* stimulating.

Safer Turns Me On

It's Hot, it's Sexy, and it's Sa . . . Uh-oh, *safer* may blow this whole project. *Safer* sounds too . . . safe. Sex means wild, uninhibited, adventurous, spontaneous, dangerous, who-gives-a-shit fun. For many of us, the less we know about someone, the more exciting it seems. Safer is for kids, medication, Volvos. Safer isn't fun, it's not real sex. So the story goes. Okay, back to Webster. "Healthy, freed or freer from harm or risk; secure from threat or danger, harm or loss; unlikely to produce controversy or contradiction; successful in reaching base in a baseball game." I like the picture of successfully reaching base. Getting to where you want to go without harm: sounds like safer sex to me!

"Unlikely to produce contradiction" is another great part of the definition, because unsafe sex is filled with contradictions, myths, misconceptions, and out-and-out lies. We've settled for sex that:

- Can infect one or both partners with nasty microorganisms (*Wild!*)
- Allows only one partner to have an orgasm (*Groovy!*)

- Makes us feel lousy emotionally and spiritually (*Fun!*)
- Is based on incorrect information or none at all (*Exciting!*)
- Produces more guilt than pleasure (*Oohwee!*)
- Tears down self-confidence and self-worth instead of building it up (*Sexy!*)
- Is sometimes violent, insensitive, hurtful, or used for emotional blackmail or an ego boost (*Thrilling!*)
- Smells bad, tastes bad, and feels bad (*Crazy!*)
- Inhibits instead of inspires (*Cool!*)
- Narrows our choices instead of expanding them (*Yow!*)
- Does everything but make us feel secure, safe, and happy (*Madness!*)

I know some people think that the word *safer* is a turn-off to sex. I've thought about that a lot, and I realized that whenever I did my best or felt the best, or had the best sex, I was feeling wonderfully safe.

Unsafe Slopes

I remember the first time I went skiing. When I perform onstage for thousands of people, I actually feel safer than I did on that mountain. I have more confidence in my skill as a performer than as a skier, and I have more knowledge about and experience in performing than I do skiing. Hence I feel safer. When I get more experience skiing, I'll probably feel safer on the mountain than I do now.

Let's apply the same logic to sex. How safe do most of us feel the first time we try sex? I say "try," because a lot of us don't do very well the first time, whether it's anal, vaginal, or oral sex.

Safe Sex or Safer Sex?

Some people say there's no such thing as *safe sex*. Wrong. Their definition of sex is too restrictive. Totally safe sex is when you have sex with yourself! I like to call it self-satisfaction! Now, don't put it down! This is a great sexual experience. Safe sex, or self-satisfaction, means you'll never reject yourself, you'll never fall asleep on yourself, and you can't give yourself anything (like a sexually transmitted disease) but a smile. So, safe sex is a great choice. *Safer sex* is when you have a sexual experience with someone else and you use something or do something that *lowers* the risk of pregnancy and of transmitting or getting an STD. Every trace of risk can't be removed from sexual activity that involves two people.

We start out having sex in notoriously unsafe spots. A backseat of a car on a wooded back road. Behind the abandoned gas station at the far end of a deserted Main Street. Harsh lighting, or none at all; it's too hot; it's too cold; knees in your throat; cramps in your legs; clothes wrapped like mummy bandages that restrict movement and reduce pleasure; and the constant threat of an audience showing up or a visit from uniformed members of the coitus-interruptus gang! Factor in all the mixed-up emotions that everyone feels the first time:

- fear of pain
- embarrassment about bodies
- worry about inexperience
- shame about premature performance
- anxiety about not knowing how to find and/or recognize an orgasm

- the stress of trying to fake sexual excitement and orgasm

Not the optimum conditions for a mutually satisfying sexual exchange. All the while our minds speak to us.

"Where is it?"

"Ugh, it's gross."

"It's slippery."

"It's hairy."

"It's moving on its own power!"

"It's too tight."

"He's heavy."

"Am I going to fart?"

No one feels safe in that sort of situation, and that's because we have it all backward. "Parking" (having sex in a car) should be tried only by experienced partners who feel very comfortable and safe with each other and know what they're doing; couples who will think it's funny if they're caught in the act. Couples who, because of their commitment to each other, can use the risky circumstances to their advantage and add sexual excitement. Couples who have dealt with all the other worries and won't be upset if an officer taps on their window! Grandparents should be the ones groping each other in the backseat! These couples feel safe and confident with each other. They are professional Hot, Sexy and Safer partners.

Hot, Sexy and Safer is a new definition of sex—a new attitude that celebrates positive male and female sexuality and sexual orientation. Safer sex *is* better sex.

3

How We View Our Private Parts

Babies discover their private parts with a total lack of embarrassment. But most parents can't deal honestly with their own sexuality, so they stop this universal form of infant play. Parents love it when their kids master figure eights on ice, for example, but when their child shows signs of acquiring physical skills for another reason, such as self-induced pleasure, they freak.

Despite discouragement from their parents, somehow guys get to know their private parts intimately anyhow—thanks to a basic male advantage. They can view theirs anytime they want. And they do! Most guys view their equipment at least four times a day—three times when they pee and one time just to admire what they've got. In fact, guys know their private parts so well that if we took Polaroids and put the photos on the wall with a hundred others, not a single guy would have trouble picking out his own. "There's mine! 'Ralphie!' The one that curves to the left!"

Women aren't made that way. It's hard for us to view our private parts. Many of us believe that only a contortionist can see what she's got. Not true. Since the invention of the hand mirror, millions of women have discovered that

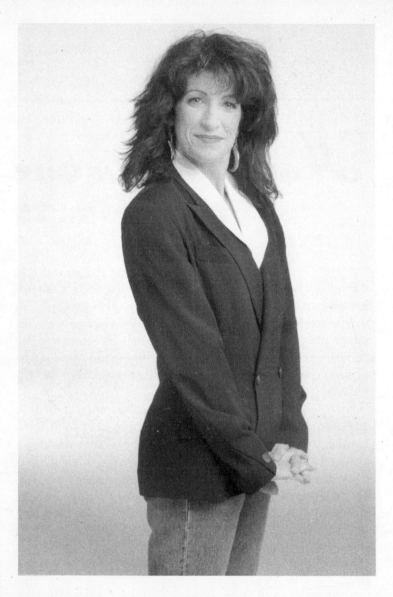

The clitoris has replaced the diamond as a girl's best friend.

they too have private parts. But to look at them and face the emotions that come with that simple act—that's scary.

Women don't like to view their private parts. It's embarrassing. We're brought up that way. Men are luckier. They grow up getting a kind of football coach's locker room speech from the world:

> Okay, gentlemen. Listen up. Your unit is the most important thing you'll ever own. Besides your car. Got that? You can walk around and hold Ralphie all day. You can show it to people. It was put on your body for pleasure, so go out and use it.

Guys believe that male private parts in general are wonderful, although lots of them worry that somehow they got issued an unusually skimpy set. On the other hand, women hear that *all* of their private parts are somehow creepy:

> Yes, you have private parts, too. But they're gross. Sorry, dears. Don't look at them and don't ever touch them. They're icky and besides, they aren't really yours. They were put on your body for someone else to use. So just wait; eventually someone will ask to use them!

Gross, Not Gross

This is nuts. We want *everyone* to practice safe sex, but half the population believes that their private parts are gross. They've inherited the idea that they don't even own them. One thing I know for sure, if we want people to change their behavior and practice safer sex, we have to change their harmful attitudes first.

You guys don't need to like your private parts less. Go ahead. Grab 'em. Admire 'em. Name 'em. We women need to like our private parts more. We need to be aware that we were brought up to dislike our own bodies. That we let others use our private parts before we do. That we allow sexist beliefs to govern our sexuality and sense of self-worth. When men owned women literally, they owned our private parts, too. Even though we are no longer chattel, women still get the message that our private parts matter less than men's. Too many women still feel like sexually inferior beings, put here to service men. Women won't make better choices about sexuality until they believe they own their own private parts.

As men and women together, we need to change how we view our private parts. Men: Make sure you're not buying the entitlement line. You're not entitled to anyone's body for your own satisfaction. Women: We must take a good, long look at our private parts before we let anyone else take a look at them. We should know them so well that we could pick them out of a crowd.

Neat, Huh?

The first thing we women need to notice is that our private parts are anything but gross. Beautiful and unique, no two alike. They're all tucked up inside, nice and neat. Nothing hangs down like on some people I know. No turkey neck skin. No fuzzy dice. Just nice, neat, smooth folds of skin for us. Look, if a male's private parts aren't gross, then neither are a female's! Believing in grossness only makes us feel gross, insecure, and less confident.

If a man's private parts are put on his body for his pleasure, the same goes for a woman and her parts. Our parts were put on our bodies for *us*—for *our* pleasure. Ours to use and enjoy. Ours to care for. Ours to be proud of. Ours to control. If we want to share them, we will—but on our terms. We don't owe our parts to anyone, and no one, *no one*, is entitled to them. What we think of our genitalia matters as much as what we think of any aspect of ourselves. When we value something, we tend to take better care of it. Women, take a good, long look at your private parts. Go ahead, do it now. (You can read the rest later. I can wait.)

What did I tell you? You have *fabulous* private parts.

For pages now, I've been referring to genitalia as private parts. That's probably silly, since so many people have made them *public parts*! Above all, I've learned one essential fact about parts. Parts don't work unless they are connected to a whole—a whole person.

So let's add another body part to the parts already mentioned: the head. Our heads have more to do with how we experience sex than any other body part. And it's not enough to know that a sperm meets an egg in one fallopian tube or the other. Sexual plumbing lectures do nothing to change sexual attitudes, which began forming when we were in diapers.

Before we learn more about our bodies, we need specific words for our genitalia. In fact, I like the word *genitalia*, except it sounds like an Italian liqueur. "Okay, that's one Drambuie, one Courvoisier, and one Genitalia. Do you want that on the rocks or straight up?"

"Yo, Melvin"

Guys, you have so many words for your parts, maybe because you're always talking to them. "Yo, Melvin, what up?" But in a book like this, I want to use mature and sophisticated words. Like Mr. Lucky Dog. El Shlongo. The one-eyed snake. Or wiener. Now *that's* sophisticated! In fact, it really doesn't matter what word I use, as long as you picture one penis and two testicles, or if you prefer, balls.

And when I talk about women's parts, I'll use "nunu!" I always like that better than most words used for women's parts: pussy, bush, vulva, beaver, bearded clam, fur burger pie. For nunu, picture our . . . wait, there's a major problem here. Society acts as if women have one private part and one only. *One*: the vagina. That's it! Just our vaginas. Nothing else is even mentioned. It's like "If you are talking about women, all you need to mention is the vagina. That makes it simple." But we have another private part, and this part is just as important, if not *more* important, than the vagina.

V.I.P. (Very Important Part)

The clitoris has been ignored for so long that people don't even agree on how to pronounce it. One way is "**klit** er us," but mine doesn't look like a "**klit** er us," so I say "kli **tor** is." Say it out loud: "**Clitoris!** I have a clitoris!" Put down the book, call up a friend, and say, "I have a clitoris." Sounds like a dinosaur. "Wow! Did you see all the Clitorises in *Jurassic Park*?" I like that, because it makes a clitoris sound big and important. Well, big it's not. But important: like you wouldn't believe.

Say "Hi!" to Your Clitoris

It's called the clitoris. Our pleasure center. The hard drive of our sexual excitement. The home of our orgasm. This shouldn't be news at the end of the twentieth century, but for many it is. No one ever sits women down and tells us where our orgasms are. Unlike men who never doubt that theirs shoot out of their wieners, we have to guess where in our bodies they take place—and how do we find them? If you ask most women where their orgasm is, you'll hear some interesting answers.

"My what? Wait—I'm so embarrassed. Oh—I know. I just read about this in *Cosmo*. Our orgasms are waiting inside of our vaginas for the big wieners from the sky to come down and release them!" If most women and men think our orgasms occur in some obscure place deep inside the vagina, it's no wonder women panic the first time they have intercourse.

("Oh my, there seems to be a whozis in my whatzis right now . . . and he's moving it back and forth, back and forth, back and forth. Look at his face—it looks like he's going to explode, and I don't feel anything! Oh no, I must be broken! I don't want him to think I'm broken, so I'll just do everything he does, and he won't know the difference. Okay, what's he doing now? He's making a pretty ugly face, and now he's making a noise!") He: "uhn." She: "aahn." He: "UHN." She: "aaahn." He: "UHNNN!" She: "AAAAAHHHHN!" ("I hope he believed that; I'm trying as hard as I can!")

Sky Wiener Not Needed

Women think they're broken because they've been given misinformation about how they work. Let's just set the record straight once and for all. Women are not broken! And *orgasms are not waiting inside of our vaginas for the big wiener from the sky to come down and release them.*

Our orgasms are, always have been, and forever will be in the clitoris.

This fact changes all the rules! It means that our orgasms are on the outside of our bodies, not on the inside! The same as a guy's. The vagina doesn't play a big role, because most positions of intercourse will never bring most women to orgasm! That's because in plain old intercourse, the clitoris is not touched, rubbed, or stimulated. Some positions encourage clitoral stimulation, but all women, like men, are built differently. Some vaginas are tilted; some clitorises are farther to the front or farther to the back, and pubic bones either protrude or recede, inhibiting or encouraging more clitoral contact.

Now for more good news: All women are capable of orgasm. True, feelings of embarrassment and shame can easily override the clitoris's ability to bring satisfaction. But when we believe we deserve orgasms, we feel the most clitoral excitement. It comes through our hearts and minds, then goes between our thighs.

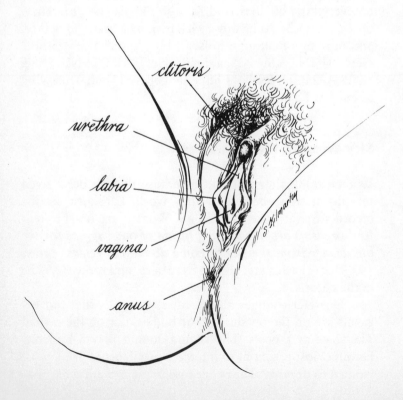

The Landolphi Theory

Some people can't deal with the fact that a woman's orgasm takes place outside her vagina. In the 1970's a Dr. Grafenberg told the world that orgasms did indeed occur inside the vagina, and he had pinpointed the very spot. As boldly as any explorer planting his nation's flag on newly discovered territory, he named the orgasm zone for himself: the notorious "G spot."

The term itself makes it sound so tiny, hidden so deep in the vagina, that it could take years to find. Maybe some women won't even take the time or trouble to find it. The idea that our orgasms depend on some minuscule spot hidden way inside of us is just another setup for failure. To me this sounds like more bunk to convince us that we have to find a bigger, longer wiener to reach this spot if we really want to have sexual satisfaction.

I have a theory I'd like to share: my commonsense approach to the "G spot" debate. First of all, early in the life of a human embryo, the area where the genitals will grow is the same for male and female. Early on in our development, the areas differentiate. A boy grows a penis and testicles, and a girl grows a clitoris and vagina. Sure, these parts look different, but I believe that they're not so different in their function and sensation. Most men agree that the end of their penis is more sensitive than the base. As the man gets more aroused, sensitivity travels down the penis and radiates to the testicles and even the anal area. It doesn't happen vice versa. The male sensation radiates from the end of the penis down to include the entire genital area.

Instead of trying to convince women that their greatest sensation is in the vagina, as the "G spot" proponents do, I see the clitoris as functioning in the same way as the penis (specifically the tip of the penis), radiating sensation. When stimulated by touching, the pleasurable sensations start to radiate along the nerve endings of the clitoris, sensitizing the vulva, the labia, and then the opening of the vagina. As the clitoris gets more stimulated, the pleasure travels into the vagina and sensitizes the inside walls of the vagina. Eventually it reaches the "G spot." I've tried rubbing that "G spot" first, before I feel aroused, and I have felt sensations, but not enough of them to have an orgasm. But the clitoris theory really works for me. Once my whole genital area is stimulated and my clitoris is erect and on the edge of releasing my orgasm, my vagina and the front inside wall can take over and bring me to orgasm.

As for the vagina, all women's vaginas have sensations, some pleasurable, some not. Every woman is unique, and every woman's vaginal sensation is unique to some degree. A vagina is very sensitive to stimulation at the opening and inside to about the first two inches. Guys who like to put their wieners in nunus should take note. Don't fret about wiener size. Two inches are as satisfying as ten inches. Many guys try to drill themselves into geological sites yet undiscovered. Don't bother.

The clitoris has all the power necessary to make a woman explode with pleasure. And, remember—it may be a private part, but it's not in hiding: the clitoris is on the *outside*.

Perpetual Show and Tell—A Note for Men

A lot of men suffer from a syndrome I call "perpetual show and tell." Most of the time, they're showing off and telling more than they're actually doing. If a guy wants to brag about sexual conquest, there ought to be a law that gives his partner equal time to relate her version.

Men in groups have a tendency to reinforce each

other's worst traits, bringing down their maturity quotient dramatically. Not only will men portray themselves as conquering sexual heroes of the locker room, but this kind of groupthink, at its extreme, can lead to sexual harassment or even gang rape. As far as sexual harassment and violence are concerned, men need to constantly remind each other that there is *never* an excuse to force any sexual experience on another person.

Men also need to change their language when talking about sex and women. Phrases like *Did you get any? Did you do her?* and *Did you score?* promote the concept of sex as a hunt or as coercion, a contest, as an I-win-she-loses situation. Other phrases that perpetuate lousy sex experiences are: Did you get laid? Did you screw, pump, bang, tag or ride her?

Men have no special rights; no entitlements. All men who coach, advise or guide groups of boys or young men are responsible for helping to create a new environment that won't accept sexist words or behavior. They need to lay down laws that clearly state a no-tolerance policy for any "group bully" tactics.

This is not to say that men are inherently evil or that they're born rapists. They're not. They have been taught to rape through their own rape, sexual abuse, or emotional abuse as children. Unfortunately, men aren't usually encouraged to remember their childhood abuse, sexual or nonsexual. They must acknowledge that it happened and talk to someone about it. Just as women are encouraged to come forward and get help for the trauma of their abuse, we must encourage our men to come forward as well. They may be walking time bombs, waiting to pass their hurt, anger, and violence on to a new victim. Not all abused men will rape, but too many will end up victimizing someone else while trying to rid themselves of hidden pain.

If men are encouraged by both their male friends and their partners to talk about their pain and fear and frailties, perhaps they won't feel compelled to become the powerful, controlling, dominant studs they hear so much about from the other guys. Men who talk and act tough are usually hiding something very soft and painful inside.

$\mathcal{S}$ex: The Wrong Way

I just finished what was probably about my five hundredth performance of Hot, Sexy and Safer. I'm sweaty—soaking wet. My leather jacket pushes down on my shoulders, making me feel extra tired and weak. No lovemaking I've ever done has been this strenuous. But unlike some sexual experiences, no one here fell asleep or left before I finished. They all stayed, gave me a standing O, and are now coming up to me throwing their arms around me, thanking me. I still think of myself as this skinny Italian girl from Beverly, Massachusetts. But they don't. They come up to me happy, surprised, inspired, thoughtful, grateful. One guy, around nineteen or twenty, fraternity sweatshirt, alpha something, baseball cap, sparse stubble, smiling, excited. "It made me think! You were so funny! You're older than my mom! I can't believe it! I never thought about, you know, sex that way, you know." Behind him is hip-hop urbanite dressed in rags and beads, with short, twisted locks sprouting only on top of his head. "It was cool, you're all right. It was dope. Thanks." Fifty more in all shapes, colors, genders, sexual orientations. I sign two more autographs. I'm beat. I start to leave, happy to go back to whatever hotel I'm in tonight. I'll never remember the room number—216? No, that was last night.

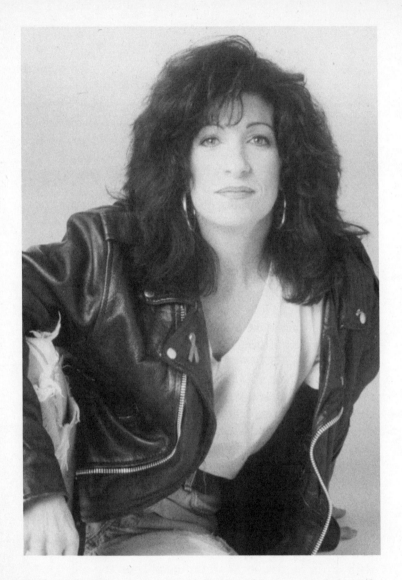

Truly great spontaneous sexual experiences are created through careful planning, discussion, and readily available safety equipment.

Then I catch this girl out of the corner of my eye. She's almost nondescript. Brown hair, brown eyes, medium height. Her clothes are neutral—there to cover, not to impress.

"Can I talk to you for a moment? If you have to leave, I understand."

"Sure." I can hardly hear her, so I move closer.

"I just wanted to tell you"—her eyes lower—"that I . . . you were great . . . I felt . . . you made me feel . . ."

I lift her chin because her words are cracking, breaking up like a bad telephone connection. Her eyes are filled with tears and spill over just as they meet mine. She's embarrassed.

"I'm sorry."

"For what?"

I know what's wrong. I don't know how I know. I wish I didn't know. I hate knowing these things. I hug her, but the feelings have already escaped.

"I know," I say to her. "It hurts. It's not fair. It's hard to think about ever trusting or feeling good about yourself, a relationship, or sex again. I know. I've been there, too!"

I was attacked when I was ten years old. It hurt. I healed. I'm happy. I have a relationship, and I feel great about me and sex.

She lifts up her head this time. I smile. Her smile forces the last two tears to stop halfway down her cheeks. I hug her and remind her that the more you cry, the less you have to pee. She thanks me and I watch her walk away.

My Story

I remember. It's been over thirty-three years since that awful night in the bunk of the cabin cruiser. I loved John like a father, a brother, a boyfriend. He was the most handsome, wonderful man I had ever met. He lived downstairs from us with two other guys. They had a lot of parties and friends over, and I could hear them in my bedroom through the hot air grate in the floor. He and his girlfriend took me to stock car races and out to dinner. My mom loved him like a son. He would stumble upstairs in the morning—usually hungover but always smiling. He'd have coffee and breakfast with us and tell us about the funny things that happened the night before. He did a lot of nice things for my mom and us three kids, like getting our car fixed or repairing things around the apartment. We were always scraping to make ends meet, and John knew it was tough on my mom.

One morning the landlord was harassing my mom for more rent when John came upstairs for a cup of coffee. The landlord looked like a bald troll next to John's six-foot-four muscular build. John backed him up against the wall and picked him up by his jacket lapels so he could look him in the eyes. He didn't say much between swears, but the landlord knew that he would be getting less rent until he fixed the old heating system. I can't remember if John carried him or threw him down the stairs.

That summer John bought a cabin cruiser, and we spent many nights sleeping on the boat while it was tied up to his friends' boats off the shore of Misery Island. The kids could run from boat to boat, diving off the bows and swimming to shore while the adults drank and ate lobster.

Violated

I slept on a wedge-shaped cushion that fit between the two beds in the bow of the boat. Nancy, John's girlfriend, was on the left, and John was on the right. Late one night I woke up as Nancy stumbled down the stairs drunk and crawled into her bunk. Even later, John returned from a late-night lobster trap raid. I was half awake and could smell seawater and beer. I felt a cold hand on my stomach. It happened so fast—no sound—I was just pulled over to his side. He was so strong; not violent, but as persistent as any drunk person can be. I had only two hands—it seemed as though he had eight or ten. At first I felt disbelief, then hurt, both physical and emotional. My heart broke that night. Not him, not him, oh God, not him. I fought as long as I could. Thank God the alcohol slowed him down. He put his fingers in me, and I felt like I was a puppet—he had all the control. My mind flooded with terror, not about what was happening, but what could or would happen after. If I scream, Nancy might wake up; she's only three feet away, she would go crazy, wake up everyone else, all the boats, tell everyone, leave him, hate him, and her heart would be broken, too.

She'd tell my mother. My mom would be devastated, hurt, she'd tell the police and he'd go to jail. Some people might not believe me, maybe it's my fault, my sister would call me stupid like she always did. Don't scream, don't scream. My two small hands gripped around his wrist—my fingers didn't even touch—pushing it back, holding on so he wouldn't go in so far and puncture my heart. Thank God the alcohol won. It killed his erection that was now trying to bulldoze my skin apart, and he collapsed half on top of me, dead weight smothering a dead little body whose heart had stopped. I remember the lack of feeling more than the pain. I thought I was dying. I thought I was dead. I felt nothing. I was numb from the inside out. I was different; the world was different; my dreams and hopes and little girl thoughts must have run out of me, or he pulled them out with his fingers and kept them with him.

Nancy, in her drunken numbness, never woke up. Twenty years later she died never knowing. John acted like nothing ever happened; maybe to him it was nothing. I didn't tell my mother until I was the mother of a little girl. She cried. She felt so bad that she didn't see it coming and couldn't protect me. I told her that I was fine and that I could heal from this. I *was* healing. I had trouble trusting and feeling safe. I know that those were the big repercussions. By then, I was learning to enjoy sex and love together. I'm still learning. It works, this healing, this lifelong healing. He didn't take my hopes and dreams. I will have them until I die. I have them here right now, and I want to share them with you to use for your own learning, healing, dreaming and hoping.

A Triumph for Me

Performing Hot, Sexy and Safer is a personal triumph for me, in several ways. First and foremost, it has helped me become sexually proud and confident. I am in charge of my sexuality and never have to prove it or use it in any negative or destructive way. Second, I am doing something I love and am proud of for my life's work and community service. My job is my service, and I don't have to compromise my happiness or my values to make a living. Third, I have created something that others can use for their own growth and betterment. It's a nonpolluting, low-maintenance, energy-producing industry that people can pass on like a chain letter. It stimulates new thoughts, attitudes, and actions and definitely creates dialogue—often where there was none before. Last, it's a lesson in empowerment for women and enlightenment for men; validation for sexual orientation; and an opportunity for society to get over its preadolescent sexual ignorance and immaturity. Hot, Sexy and Safer isn't me—it's everyone who has participated and walked away saying, "Gee, I never thought about it that way."

5

*M*e and My Genitals

Our parents tell us to become independent, self-sufficient, and assertive. We're told: "Take matters into your own hands." I totally agree! Take matters into your own hands: masturbate!

Baby girls and baby boys enjoy touching themselves. Touching feels good and comforting. Girls don't walk around holding on to themselves as much as boys do, probably because they don't have a convenient handle. But if you watch little girls, you'll see that they sit with their hands between their legs while listening to stories or watching TV, and they slide up and down the jungle gym looking for the "good feeling."

It Feels Good

Little boys and girls tell us about good feelings quite openly. They don't obsess about them or put much importance on them. The good feelings are just plain fun. If there's a problem with their penis or vulva, they'll show it to you or ask if you can see what's causing the itch or irritation. No embarrassment, no judgment.

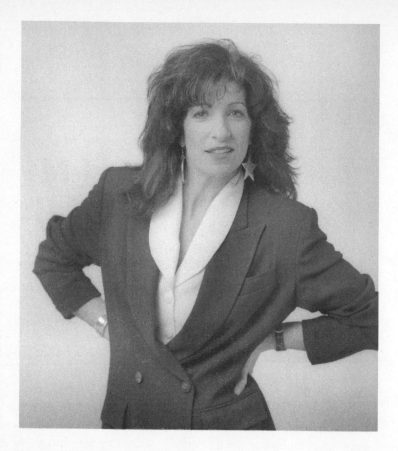

If you haven't discovered your own private parts, don't play with someone else's.

But as we grow up, we start to get some strong messages about touching our private parts. Rather than learning that masturbation can be a safe, healthy, and enjoyable form of sexual expression, we hear a lot of different versions of "Don't do it." *You'll break it, you'll go blind, it's dirty.* A few more enlightened parents may tell you to do it in your room with the door locked and don't do it too much. No one says what "too much" is and what the consequences would be.

Don't Forget to Eat

Too much would be losing interest in everything else, including food.

When we masturbate we touch ourselves and excite our genitals, usually to orgasm. Simple, clear. No biggie. Yet the topic of masturbation causes more embarrassment than any other sexual issue except anal intercourse. Strange. Getting naked with another person (maybe one we don't even know) and putting our genitals together, licking them, touching them, and swapping body fluids and germs—that should feel much more embarrassing than touching our own parts. I don't get it.

If we wanted to, we could look at masturbating in a different way. A simple attitude change could make us feel better about taking care of ourselves sexually. Instead of considering masturbation a perverse and antispiritual, male-only entitlement and health necessity, we could take a more positive, commonsense approach to self-satisfaction.

Self-Love

When sex therapists and sex educators talk about sex— usually meaning intercourse with another person—they often stress the importance of intimacy. Intimacy means a closeness created through trust, respect, and love, a closeness that makes each person feel safe enough to share secrets, desires, thoughts and feelings, without fearing judgment and rejection. Safe enough to depend on each other for support and caring when either one is feeling scared or sad. Safe enough to express sexual pleasure and passion, to be physically, emotionally, and spiritually naked. Through masturbation we can learn a similar kind of intimacy with ourselves.

Masturbation has come to be thought of as a purely selfish act done by those who are oversexed and unable to control their sexual urges or who are too ugly to attract a partner. For women, masturbation is supposed to be especially dirty and gross. Some religions preach that masturbation only leads to further evil sexual behavior. This, most certainly, has never been proven! In fact, the denial of sexual expression can be *more* emotionally dangerous and leave people feeling *less* in control.

Common sense tells us to be intimate with ourselves before we connect with someone else. Until I trust, love, and respect myself, including my genitals, I can't believe that someone else does. If I treat my genitals with fear and loathing, there's a good chance I'll let others treat me the same way. Masturbating is a way of showing that we like and take care of ourselves.

Masturbating:

- releases tension
- helps to alleviate headaches, even migraines
- releases endorphins in the body, which trigger happy, contented feelings

- helps circulate blood flow, especially in the genital area
- teaches us how to have an orgasm
- encourages self-love and self-care
- helps make sexual expression a healthy part of life
- (with a partner) is a great alternative to intercourse
- helps us get to know our own bodies

I like the expression *self-satisfaction* better than *masturbation*. It sounds more positive and doesn't focus on just genital stimulation. When we feel satisfied, we don't feel anxious, tense, afraid, sad, depressed, angry, guilty, or hurt. If we changed our attitudes about masturbating, we'd get more positive results from doing it. Masturbation is a step in the process of sexual growth, a natural form of sexual expression.

How to have better self-satisfaction experiences:

1. Explore where you got your ideas and beliefs about masturbation, and question their validity.
2. Find a comfortable, private place.
3. Use pictures, videos, books to help, if you want to. (Be careful not to get so dependent on these that you can't masturbate without them or with someone you care about.)
4. Go slowly and be gentle with yourself.
5. Use a vibrator if you want. (Again, make sure you can achieve orgasm without using it, too.)
6. Fantasize. (Don't make moral judgments about your fantasies—they are make-believe, not what you would necessarily do in real life.)
7. Don't make masturbation work; it's fun. Learn to "play" with yourself.

8. Ask friends and people you love, trust, and respect how they feel about masturbation.
9. Never lie about your masturbation habits.
10. If you feel guilty or out of control, talk to a counselor and tell the truth.
11. Work on loving and feeling proud of yourself and your body.
12. Don't masturbate while using drugs or alcohol— they don't help, and they make it more difficult to reach orgasm.
13. Don't masturbate with objects that can hurt you, cut you, or get lost in you.
14. Remember, billions of people have masturbated.
15. Masturbate with a sense of humor.
16. Read other sex books and their ideas on masturbation. Try to find books and ideas that celebrate your sexual orientation and do not degrade or abuse either gender or any race.

6

*L*earning to Masturbate, Again!

At twenty-six I realized something that startled me: I had lost the ability to masturbate. Something I could do at four, I couldn't do as a grown woman. My marriage had ended a year or two before, and I remember now exactly what it was like to learn again how to give myself pleasure . . .

I'm embarrassed in front of myself! How can that be? Here I am, lying in bed, in the dark, the covers up to my neck, not knowing where to start. How is it that my ex-husband—who I don't even like or feel comfortable with anymore—knows how to touch me better than I do myself? After all, this is my body. But, I'm trying to use common sense. Maybe if I pretend I'm someone else touching me, I'll feel less embarrassed.

That helps. I fantasize about someone stroking me gently. Good, but then I hear something that distracts me—my baby daughter in the next room. My daughter! What would she think of her mother masturbating? Somehow, motherhood and masturbation have never occupied my mind at the same moment before. I come from a culture in which motherhood and sexuality don't meet. For a lot of women, trying to balance the two and enjoy them both is almost impossible.

Men don't seem to have a problem being sexual and

being a parent. Now I'm pissed. I bet my ex-husband is masturbating right now and enjoying it, and I'm here struggling. Okay, that's it. Now I'm going for it. I deserve to be sexual and to masturbate without embarrassment or guilt.

I relax and take some deep breaths. I touch myself all over with gentleness and respect. I don't just grab my crotch or breasts like a kid devouring candy. It suddenly occurs to me that there's one big advantage to masturbating. I can touch myself the way I want at the speed I want. I respond to these nice touches. Sometimes I lose my concentration, but I don't get upset. I just start again. I fantasize and keep exploring. I don't reach orgasm this first time, but I like it. I'm proud of myself. I've started to like me a little more.

Afterward I could feel my sense of independence grow, like the first time a child ties his or her own shoes. I felt like I'd climbed the tree just as good as any boy.

Each night, teasing myself and breaking down years of self-embarrassment, I got closer. Then one night, I did it. I felt all the shouldn'ts and don'ts, which had blackmailed me as a girl, squeeze out of my genitals with each contraction of my orgasm! I enjoyed my genitals. I gave myself pleasure. I liked touching me and feeling my body and its juice. I squeezed juice. I created sweat. A feeling of contentment flowed from within me.

If men can love their sex, so can I. If they can enjoy masturbating, so can I. If they can take care of themselves, so can I. Motherhood and masturbation go great together.

So I learned how to masturbate. Got real good at it, too. Now I find that sometimes I simply feel like giving myself pleasure.

Flying Solo

Sometimes I need two orgasms. He's sleeping next to me, and we both had one each, together. But I can't sleep, and I'd like another orgasm. I could wake him up, but I don't need to, nor do I really want to. I don't want to make love or have intercourse again. I just want another orgasm.

I can remember when I felt guilty long ago about masturbating while my partner slept, because I'd faked my earlier orgasm. I never fake orgasms now. I just want another one—all by myself, without guilt.

It's not that I lack great sex: we have *that*. My own orgasm is just something extra. He can sleep and I can have another orgasm. He can snore a little and I can moan a little. Sounds fair to me. This one has certain qualities that make it more . . . personal: more of a total body orgasm, too.

Totally Tense

I have to tense up every muscle, *every* muscle, and rub my clitoris very fast and hard until my finger, wrist, then my whole arm goes numb. I stop and start at least three times because I get so tired just before I "fall off the edge." My head pounds as hard while I'm trying to have "it" as when I do have "it." My teeth clench, too! Maybe this kind of O is made up of tension that builds up over the weeks and can get "flushed" only with this kind of intensity. I don't have a lot of different kinds of orgasms, but this one has a distinctive quality, and I like it. I know it and I enjoy its mad, funny ways.

I'll tell him in the morning. He'll say, "Why didn't you wake me?" and I'll say, "This one's for me."

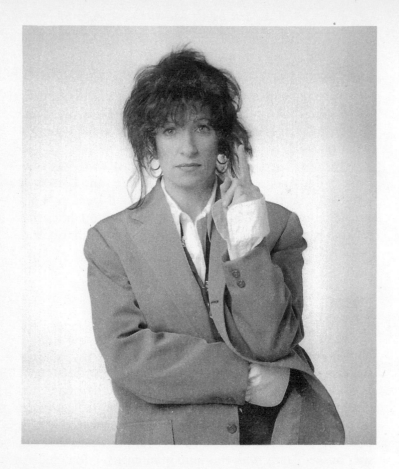

Even though I helped to create an erection, it's not my job to fix it.

7

*M*y Life with Erections

Having an erection must really be an experience. Yikes! I can't even imagine having a part of me twitch, shudder, and slowly start to rise, defying gravity like some special effect in a Japanese horror flick. An erection does look as if you're supposed to do something with it. But sometimes what you have to do with it is leave it alone.

Maybe this event called an erection gets too much respect. I don't know why. To me, it seems so mechanical. A penis goes erect and a little buzzer sounds with a flashing sign: "Erection complete. Time for intercourse."

Most guys get hard-ons day and night. They could open a store and call it "Boners R Us." Washing a penis can start one. Walking in tight jeans, walking in loose jeans, watching TV, reading, chewing gum, dancing, kissing, bowling, doing karate, a strong wind—look, it happened again!

All Eyes on Woodrow

Here we are making out, feeling around, things are heating up when . . . he gets an erection. Okay, everything shifts gears—now the focus is on his woody! Simply because it's there, because we can both see it, he's proud of it, and it looks like it needs fixing. A woody feels like it's supposed to do something. "If I have one, I shouldn't let it go to waste, right?"

Suddenly the woman feels she's at a distinct disadvantage. She doesn't have an inflatable appendage to wave around like a baseball bat, so she seems less important. Plus, she has a place for him to put his erection. He knows that, and she knows that. But that doesn't mean his erection *has* to go in there.

What if we looked at an erection more like a stick shift? Something to grab on to and wrestle 'til it pops. You can pull it, stroke it, wiggle it, hang things on it! Shift it to first, second, third, and fourth, even overdrive to fifth (forget reverse).

Brain Erections

I have a friend, a dear, dear friend, who lives in a wheelchair. Since he's paralyzed below the waist, he doesn't get erections, but he says that he has "psych"asms instead of orgasms. They originate in his mind, not his penis. I believe he feels these. I've even experienced them with him. He definitely felt and had a "gasm" of some kind. All erections really start in the brain. They just end up showing themselves in the penis. My friend's psychasms may even be better than the conventional variety, because they take place closer to the source.

As a woman who has experienced erections up close and personal, I can say that as neat as they are—and they certainly can give pleasure—if the man I loved couldn't get one, I wouldn't feel like I was missing a lot. Hands and fingers stay hard longer, much longer, and have more dexterity. Objects shaped like penises can be used with great effectiveness and finesse; some of them even vibrate. Soon they'll even talk: "Just because I'm plastic you think you don't have to respect me."

No one erection is more important than my safety, self-worth, and well-being. Men will have thousands of erections in their lives; not all of them have to be cared for or taken too seriously.

Enlightened Teen

Luckily sometimes you run into men who don't try to rule the world with their penises. I had the good fortune of picking a remarkably enlightened teenager as my first boyfriend, Jimmy. The first erection I ever felt belonged to him. Prone together on my couch. I thought, "belt buckle?" Then "definitely *not* belt buckle." I can remember my surprise at its hardness. All at once, I understood the word *boner*.

I wondered if it hurt him when we would grind our pelvises together. It hurt my pelvic bone sometimes if we pressed too hard for too long. Terminally shy, we never talked about these erections, and for over a year, I only felt it through our clothes. Sometimes he would rearrange it. I wondered if it would break if it got bent too much. But it never broke, no matter how hard we pressed on it. His erection was present whenever we made out.

Soft and Hard

After a year, I got to touch it with my hand. Never saw it, just touched it. First through his jeans or chinos. I remember rubbing his chest and stomach, and in each session, I moved my hand a little lower. For weeks, I stayed at the belt buckle, the border between me and it. But eventually that buckle lost its significance, and one night my hand jumped the fence and traveled down over the zipper until I felt what my pelvic bone had been sliding on for so long. I couldn't make out a lot of details through the fabric. His body was long and thin, and I wondered if his erection would be similar. It was, but later I found out that that's not generally true. Anyway, I rubbed it and then pressed on it. I could feel the softness and hardness. I could feel it grow bigger and smaller in response to my touch, and I jumped the first time that it jumped! I wondered if he could control that.

I eventually moved my hand down inside his jeans and felt my first erection in the flesh: warm, bumpy, arrow shaped, moist, and twitching a lot. Such soft skin on such a hard object! I couldn't get my entire hand around it because he still had on his jeans. We both felt content for many more months.

I'd like to point out something that may not seem obvious. Jimmy and I were having sex. Two human beings gave each other physical pleasure: sex. In my book sex and sexual intercourse are not synonymous. You can have sex with your clothes on, without sexual intercourse. (You can read more about this in chapter 19.)

See Me, Feel Me, Touch Me

With all that touching, I never actually looked at Jimmy's erection. My first erection sighting happened years later, on a snowy night in a car with an older guy. I was eighteen, and he must have been about twenty-three or twenty-four, one of those intense, young idealists—philosopher, self-styled poet, and political activist—filled with passion and anger. He loved and hated equally, and he scared the shit out of me. But he intrigued me, and he actually wanted to spend time with me! Alone.

As we parked, I tried to follow the big college words he used to express those high ideals. He was getting excited about what he was saying, or so I thought, but his excitement must have traveled to his dick. During one of his impassioned dissertations, he leaned over and kissed me. While he kissed me, he must have deftly pulled out his erection, because before I knew it, he put his very large, very hard dick in my hand. There was plenty of light in the car, and I looked down to see it. It looked so big in my small hand, and it seemed to turn purple from the pressure of his grip. I tried to pull away, but he held on like a vise. I couldn't believe it as he moved my hand up and down his erection. In four strokes, he came on me. It was warm—no, hot—and white. I watched his dick erupt all over my skin.

"Son of a bitch! How dare you do this to me!" Words came out of my mouth harder and faster than his semen did. I was so angry. All his high and mighty philosophy about life and humankind amounted to so much bullshit. He only cared about his hard-on and finding some naive sap like me to come around and listen to his crap and hold it for him. What a loser! The next time I held an erection, I did it on my own terms.

The One That Curves to the Left

When I went back to college at twenty-four after leaving a short marriage that didn't work (except that it produced my beautiful daughter), I met a fellow student named Andre. Tall, very tall, lithe, dark hair, mocha skin. I wanted him to perform with me in a duet I had choreographed. The difference in our heights would be striking. His long limbs were exactly what I'd thought of when I created the dance. He agreed.

It was a sensual dance that required intense eye and body contact. Very provocative for a private New England college where black and white met but never touched. The piece required intensity and skill. We rehearsed until we were punch-drunk. My respect for Andre grew as I experienced his tenacity. He endured unmerciful taunting from his fraternity brothers and from his black female friends. At one point in the dance, I ran to him with all my speed and jumped as he lifted me over his six-foot-five body. Sometimes we made it; most times, we didn't. The night of the performance, we made it. Everyone on campus talked about us for weeks.

The dancing brought us closer together than most friends or lovers. And one day we decided to try a new dance. No music, no choreographed routine, no clothes. I felt safe with Andre. We cared for each other. Our strong, mutual physical attraction seemed natural.

Big-Time Embarrassment

During our rehearsals, we had already touched each other in every conceivable place. I thought this new step would be easy and not embarrassing. We kissed. We touched a little bit and started to peel off our body-hugging spandex. But he stopped. The tight briefs wouldn't come off. I couldn't imagine what made him reluctant. I told him that I wasn't ready for intercourse, but that I'd love to rub and touch. He said that he felt too embarrassed. Andre?

He said that he was different. He was upset, almost crying. What had I done? What could be so different that it could cause this very confident, sensual man to be shaking with fear? I sensed it had something to do with his genitals, something he thought was too horrible for me to see. What could be so horrible? I had stretch marks from my pregnancy, cellulite, and breasts that had fed my baby daughter. My body was definitely not perfect.

A Different Kind of Guy

Because I felt so comfortable in our friendship, I sincerely convinced him that whatever was so different about his body, it was part of a person I cared about. I said I wanted him always to be proud of who he is—all of who he is. We kissed some more, and in the dim light, he took off his underwear. The penis that sprang out curved up and to the left, like a sideways question mark! This was not a subtle nuance. This was not a slight bend; this was a hairpin curve, the kind that has warning signs on a mountain road. I looked at it for a few seconds, and then I held it in both hands while I looked up at his face. Tears had collected in the corners of his eyes. I kissed his eyes and said, "I've found a man with a unique sense of direction! This will touch those hard-to-reach spots!" He and I both laughed and laughed. With a little bit of creative maneuvering and positioning, we enjoyed rubbing and touching until we were both satisfied. We then snuggled in each other's arms and talked about his uniquely curved penis, the pros and cons.

Now we were two friends discussing the solution to a problem, just like we did in our dance routine. "Well, if you enter the vagina before you're fully hard, it should be easier that way. Let the vagina straighten it out! Lie down on your right side and enter from the back. Most vaginas have some curve to them, too." Then we got silly; "Use a penis splint . . . Have her stand on her head, then rotate like a corkscrew . . . Fold it over and let it spring open once it's inside." Tears of laughter were rolling down our cheeks. I looked into his eyes and told him that he should love his uniqueness, because life was filled with the bland and boring. When life throws you a curve, learn how to use it to its fullest advantage.

Andre taught me a lot about the insecurity of men who feel sexually inadequate. Under our underwear, we are all at our most vulnerable, whether it curves to the left or not.

Mr. "I'm Doing You a Favor"

He's his own best sex partner, and watching him having intercourse with our vaginas is an experience many women share but few talk about. While lying on our backs looking up at this grimacing, sweating, uncoordinated alien lost in sex space, we watch with detached amazement as he races with himself to experience the ultimate satisfaction. Wanting to leave his mark—graffiti scribbled on the inside walls of our vaginas: "I was here, '94."

Do these men realize or even care how silly they look pumping away, fighting with their own genitals to get them there faster and better than the last time? Maybe they're thinking, "This could be the last time for a long time, so make it good!"

Sometimes they peek at us and see where we are in their frantic rush to ecstasy. They're thinking, "Are you coming with me, because I'm there and I ain't stopping! Too late!" I thought once that maybe a mirror might change this scenario. Ha! It only made things worse. They love watching themselves—can't get enough of their brilliant performances.

These men give intercourse a bad reputation. Now I can tell—before we're anywhere near the bedroom—if one of these men is going to be a selfish lover. All talk is about them, their jobs, accomplishments, interests, and needs. They have no ability to laugh at themselves. They primp a lot (or not at all) and need "things," such as cars and clothes, to enhance their image. When they move, they expect everyone to watch them—even other guys—in a nonsexual, envious way.

Thank goodness there aren't a lot of these guys.

I think it's just that they stand out and get recycled a lot because too many women get wise to their bullshit. I'm an ex-member of that sisterhood. Call me if you need to talk about Mr. "I'm Doing You a Favor." These guys are definitely easier to quit than chocolate chip cookies!

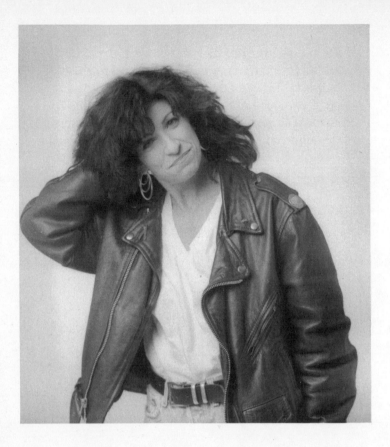

Intercourse is the easiest thing to do badly and the hardest thing to do well.

8

*I*ntercourse Can Get in the Way of Great Sex

Approximately one-third of 15-year-olds have had sexual intercourse. Thirty-two percent of females and 58 percent of males age 16, 51 percent of females and 67 percent of males age 17, and 70 percent of females and 79 percent of males age 18 report ever having sexual intercourse.

> —Advocates for Youth (formerly The Center for Population Options), *Adolescent Sexual Behavior, Pregnancy and Parenthood, Fact Sheet.* January, 1994.

"It was the worst experience of my life." I hear that all the time from young guys talking about the first time they had intercourse with a woman. For almost all of them, it was a horror show! "I thought it was going to be magic," they tell me. "It was horrible." After the experience they felt disappointed, and more, they felt embarrassed and demoralized.

"It was quick, way too quick on my part." Not surprisingly, coming too soon was one of the major reasons for embarrassment. These young men either didn't get all the way inside or didn't get in at all. Some who pushed forward before coming suffered an embarrassment they experienced as even worse—not coming at all. "I was in there for forty-five minutes," one man told me, "and she finally said, 'Are you done yet?' " Most guys didn't use a condom. Many of those who did say it came off before they finished. Sometimes broken condoms went unnoticed until after the fact.

Here's what's usually missing the first time couples try intercourse:

- light
- any sort of honest discussion
- finesse
- even one partner with self-confidence
- mutual love
- two sexually aroused partners

Add guilt, fear, strange odors and sounds, pain, embarrassment, clumsiness, the weight of expectations connected with the "first time," and anxiety that has been simmering, boiling, and open-flame broiling for roughly fourteen to twenty years. I find it astounding that anyone would go back for a second time!

Talk to Me!

Frequently first intercourse took place in physically uncomfortable locations susceptible to intruders, which added to feelings of being unsafe and needing to rush. The men had little or no knowledge of a woman's equipment, but they did have ego-wrenching pressure not to screw up, fart, or lose control. But the worst part, most men tell me, was that their partner gave no feedback or encouragement.

Usually, when you're a kid, or even when you're an adult, and you try something difficult for the first time, you get a pat on the back and some words of encouragement:

"good job," "keep trying," "you did great for your first time," "you're a real natural," "don't worry—it gets better as you practice." The first time you get laid, you won't find anyone there rooting you on. Guys who play sports come to expect cheers for their physical performance. This performance was nothing to cheer about and besides, the cheerleader just ran to the bathroom, leaving you with your pants around your ankles and a gooey penis dripping on your thigh.

Mr. Used and Abandoned

Contrary to the image I once had of young men, they experienced lack of affection as painful. They wanted cuddling. A pervasive feeling of being uncomfortable probably kept both partners from showing much emotion, but I never expected to hear about guys' deep feelings of rejection. They felt abandoned and used. Yes, *used!* They felt that they'd failed themselves and their partners. They worried that they'd hurt their partners, and they felt sorry for it. All in all, they compared their first intercourse to a plane crash onto the frozen tundra.

Worse, they couldn't admit this disaster to anyone. They told me about lying to their buddies and trying to forget what really happened. In doing so, they gained one consolation: they'd scored. In the eyes of the world, they became men.

The secrets men hide! I always thought a guy's first intercourse was great, or at least a hundred times better than mine or any other woman's. I assumed that young men just felt so relieved to have met the cultural pressure to lose their virginity that details didn't matter. I guess that society's emphasis on intercourse as an active sex act for men and a passive one for women led me to believe that guys had it easier in every way. Apparently not.

The Other Side

From a woman's perspective, of course, the first time was even worse! Many of my early experiences put me on the defensive—physically, emotionally, and spiritually. "Is he going to force himself on me and in me? Am I being used? What's going to happen tomorrow? Can I stand the guilt?" This defensiveness came from the double standard imposed on women. He hears he should go after sex and get laid; she must refuse, hold out, and wait. If society sets women up as keepers of the "prize," then society has to expect women to use their power to try to get what they want—a relationship, a commitment, the words "I love you," affection, compliments, or maybe some goal that has nothing to do with their partners, such as revenge against their parents. I never even considered some of my early partners' feelings. That seems so strange to me now.

I can almost guarantee that anyone's first experience with intercourse will be disappointing. Young people need honest information from those with healthy experiences of intercourse. I'd like to see those of us with positive sexual experiences talk to those with none long before they try it. I mean, really talk. Without bragging or throwing in personal agendas, misinformation, fear and damnation, or sexism. We would relate the experience with honest, detailed descriptions that take into account the physical, emotional, and spiritual aspects of the act.

Intercourse is something anyone can do badly and few, if any, beginners do well. This sexual act was not meant to be one of our first sexual experiences. All the stuff you see on TV and in movies is very far from reality. X-rated films don't begin to show the whole picture. To ensure a great experience for both partners, create a high level of physical, emotional, and spiritual comfort. Employ mutual respect, love, and trust. Too many people settle for less: what a shame!

This needed sense of comfort comes from honest communication, too. Tell each other what you like at the time you're doing it; let your partner know how excited you are, what's working or not working, and how close you are to orgasm. Most women will not have an orgasm through intercourse because 99% of the positions used don't even touch the clitoris. So this act will probably only satisfy one of the partners. You will need to talk to each other. Use words—not grunts, groans, and hand signals—so you can tell if your partner is truly excited and happy about the situation, or faking it. You need plenty of time in physically comfortable, private surroundings (which include a door that locks).

Don't Do *It* Until You Do *This*

Find Your Own Orgasm.   First, you should definitely know where your own orgasm is located and how to have one by yourself. (See chapter 5, Me and My Genitals.)

Instruct Your Partner.   You should be able to instruct your partner on your likes and dislikes and be able to help him or her find your pleasure areas.

Show and Tell.   You should be able to touch yourself in front of your partner. If you are too ashamed to touch your own body and help arouse yourself sexually, you're not ready for the mutual cooperation needed for intercourse. Intercourse is a true "show and tell"!

Look.   Unless you and your partner agree to do it with the lights on so that you can see minute details of each other's private parts, as well as the look in each other's eyes, you're not ready.

Get the Right Safety Gear.   Know how to use
birth control effectively and then use it. Know how
to use a condom correctly and then use it. (See
chapter 11, Condomania.)

Explore.   A man ought to put a finger gently inside
the vagina before he puts his penis in there. That
way, he can explore it, getting to know its limitations
and how it feels, and she can teach him about her
body and guide him. A woman should make sure she
puts her own finger inside herself before she lets
anyone else do it. No sharp fingernails, and always
wash your hands first.

Be 100 Percent Honest with Yourself.   Question
yourself on why you are going to participate in
intercourse, and tell yourself the truth.

Be Prepared to Change.   Intercourse affects every
part of us, from our soul to our sinuses. There is no
way you can separate your emotions from the
physical act. No way. You can pretend, but the
effects will be there.

You may be thinking, "Well, I haven't followed half of
these suggestions, and I've been having intercourse for a
long time." Okay, I've got some questions for you, and since
you're not here, I'll fill in your answers based on conversa-
tions I've had with audience members from coast to coast.

Q. Are you happy, proud, and satisfied with your intercourse experiences?
A. Well, yeah. I mean, not all the time. Sometimes. A
   few times. But no one is satisfied all the time. That's
   just the way it is.

Q. But are you ever satisfied? Are you proud of your sex life? Enough to brag about the reality, or are you lying about the fantasy?

A. I just don't expect much. I just think everyone else has great intercourse but me.

That's the problem. No one gives out the real deal about intercourse. Beginning with adults who have tons of excuses for keeping the information they have secret.

Excuse #1: "If we tell people how to do it right, especially kids, they'll just run out and do it!"

This is pure myth, not true and never has been. In fact, when kids get good information, just the opposite happens. I received graphic details about intercourse from my mom beginning when I was twelve, but I didn't have intercourse until I was twenty. I knew I wasn't ready for semen to run down my leg and all the other things I thought were gross. But I still had sex and more orgasms than my girlfriends who were "doing it," and unlike some of them, I never got pregnant or contracted an STD.

Excuse #2: "Well, that's too personal and embarrassing to talk about."

I remember when I found buying underwear in a department store too personal. God forbid a guy should walk by while I was holding up a pair of panties. I got over that embarrassment or I'd still be wearing the same panties I wore in high school! I matured: I can buy underwear in public, and I can talk about intercourse. Unless people with experience get over their embarrassment and talk honestly about sexual intercourse, attitudes won't change.

If you yourself are too embarrassed to act openly and talk honestly with your partner before you have intercourse, then forget about intercourse for now. At least delay it until you can ask yourself and then your partner why you plan to do it. I mean it. Love alone won't get you through this intense and important experience. Be honest, really honest. Tell your partner what you expect from intercourse. Be realistic. If you're lying to yourself and your partner, intercourse will only exacerbate the dishonesty.

14 Things I Want You to Know About Intercourse

1. Taking off another person's clothes is awkward and requires mutual help so sensitive body parts don't get caught in a zipper.
2. Your hair can get pulled or caught on something.
3. In most positions, your partner sees more of your genitals than you do.
4. You may find yourself in odd positions, ones that can make you feel uncomfortable and vulnerable.
5. While you're putting on a condom and inserting other birth control devices, you're dealing with each other's body smells, tastes, sweat, and other fluids and gases.
6. Be ready for noises made by body suction, vaginal suction, and farts.
7. Eventually, you have to pee.
8. You get hair from all over your bodies in your mouth.
9. Finding the right opening is confusing.
10. Trying to find a position where the penis rubs the clitoris is not only difficult but impossible for most—use your own hand to rub your clitoris during intercourse. It works.
11. Trying to find the right amount of thrust power,

upward pushing, and downward stroking, and figuring out how far you should go in takes caring and mutual concern for each other's pleasure and comfort.
12. You're not sure how fast both of you should move or when to speed up or slow down.
13. Trying to listen for intruders is distracting.
14. Trying to be quiet so your roommate, family, or friends won't hear you is certainly challenging.

Whenever we attempt something new with someone else, we use some basic commonsense guidelines. Whether we're doing this project for business, school, or for fun, we know we should be honest, cooperate, and compromise, if we need to. We try not to bully, be selfish, cheat, hurt each other, or call each other names. We try to know our duties or job responsibilities, use our equipment properly and take care of it, treat other people's equipment with respect, have a positive attitude, and smile. All these guidelines apply to intercourse.

Just to recap my thoughts about "doing it": We need a more honest picture of just what sex means. First, intercourse alone won't bring most women to orgasm. Second, it's very easy to do badly or selfishly. Finally, it's very difficult to do in a nonembarrassing, mutually satisfying way.

Most of us use the word *sex* to mean *only* intercourse. "Did you have sex with him (or her)?" That's too narrow and restricted a definition for sex. For instance, people may ask,

"Are you sexually active?"

"Yes, but I only use whipped cream and a rubber chicken."

"That's not sex!"

"Don't tell my chicken that."

But what if the answer was: Yes, I'm sexually active, but remember, there are 2,862 ways to sexually satisfy your partner and yourself without intercourse. (I know this because I'm up to 1,906!) I'm sexually active even though I'm not having intercourse, either anal or vaginal. In fact, I'm even *more* sexually active than some people who have intercourse.

Sex needs a better and more inclusive definition these days. It should include mutual touching, rubbing, licking, light chewing, whipped cream, trapezes, opened eyes, and anything else you can try or imagine.

My First Time

My first time wasn't so terrible. But, unlike most people I know, I'd done a lot of preparation for it, and I was twenty years old. We were engaged. We intended to build a life together, with children eventually. Even though I didn't want to get pregnant then, if it happened, we were prepared to love our child. I was on the pill, but I knew that I still faced some risk. No one talked about using condoms to cut down on STDs back then—we only worried about pregnancy. My boyfriend and I had had lots of sex without actually engaging in vaginal intercourse. We had orgasms. We rubbed and touched, kissed and masturbated each other. On "the big night," we talked first and took our time. I felt fairly relaxed but anxious, too. This was my first experience with intercourse, a momentous occasion, and it wasn't something done out of ignorance, fear, desperation, uncontrollable passion, or under duress or alcohol or other drugs. We fully accepted the possible ramifications of our conscious choice.

It was early spring in the mountains of New Hampshire. We walked through snow to reach the large dormitory cabin with rows and rows of cots at the outdoor education center where he worked. The kids wouldn't arrive back until summer vacation, so we had our privacy.

We chose our cot and snuggled under the starched white sheets and navy blue wool blanket. We talked and kissed and talked and rubbed and made sure both of us felt ready. When I was at my peak of sexual arousal and he was close but still able to control his explosion, we both maneuvered his penis into my vagina. It was tight, but it didn't hurt. We were both wet, and there was no need to force it. It was a strange sensation, to say the least. But not traumatic. We moved together, with me following his lead. He'd done this before, but at twenty-two, he didn't quite qualify as an expert.

I didn't know when his orgasm would happen, so I asked him to tell me. He was getting closer. I felt some sensation, but not like when I laid on top of him and slid up and down on his erection. I tried to push to get more sensation but found that being on my back wasn't the best position for my pleasure. He asked me if I was close. I could've lied or told the truth. I told the truth: I wasn't. He suggested that I get on top. So, very carefully, we changed positions. He guided himself into me while I lifted up on my knees. When I lowered myself on him and laid on top of his stomach, I knew this would work. I could feel him in me. Now I could rub my clitoris on his erection from the inside—what an amazing thing! The full moon was our guiding light as we figured out how to rock together.

Just before I exploded, I felt him get bigger, as my vagina tightened around him. Still no pain. He never pushed too hard. He never moved just for himself. He waited for me, and I felt safe. In a very shaky voice, I said I was ready, and he lifted his whole body to meet me. Ten seconds later, we collapsed, with me still on top. I felt his penis slowly slide out of me, and I looked into his eyes and smiled. It was okay—no, it was good—we did great, and the next morning I knew we would be just fine.

David's First Intercourse Experience

I think that a lot of women believe or assume that a man's first intercourse experience is much better than a woman's. At least we are led to believe that from the bravado and joking which most men convey when recounting it. I've learned through talking privately with so many young men that that wasn't necessarily the case. So, I asked my friend David if he would tell me about his first intercourse experience. Here's his recollection in his own words.

I knew I didn't know what I thought about sex. But my best friend, Rocky, a year older than me at fourteen, hatched a plan to rid me of my ignorance. Rocky knew a girl named Carla who was, for her own confused adolescent reasons, willing to correct my problem. Rocky was there only to show me the ropes. We went to Carla's house on a night her family was at a religious service. Rocky had been there before, so he knew exactly what to do. Within minutes of our sneaking in her bedroom window, Rocky was on top of her. I had been ordered to the kitchen to fix Carla a peanut butter sandwich. When I returned, Rocky was sitting half-clothed in a chair facing Carla, who was lying naked on her bed.

When I handed Carla her sandwich, Rocky handed me a condom.

"Your turn," he said as he pushed me toward the bed. This was my first chance to really look at Carla, a plain, white-skinned, rather plump sixteen-year-old.

"Come on," she said, "my parents will only be gone for an hour." She took a healthy bite of her sandwich and spread her legs.

Again Rocky pushed me toward the bed. "Don't take

off your pants, just push them down, in case we have to run out." In seconds I was kneeling over her, trying to put the condom on a totally frightened penis. Rocky, laughing at my dilemma, didn't help matters. Carla, with as much understanding of the situation as her nature would muster, placed her hand on my penis, then grabbed my left hand and plowed my two fingers into her vagina. Satisfied that she had shown me where things were, she went back to consuming her sandwich.

In seconds, my raging hormones bulldozed over my fears. As soon as the rubber was on, Rocky began barking instructions. "Lay down on her and put it in her," he shouted. "Now pump your ass in and out." Rocky's face was inches away from my point of entry.

"Here, grab her titties." Rocky's right hand squeezed and mauled a chubby breast, and as I lifted my head up, Carla was looking over to Rocky expressionless, taking another bite of her half-eaten sandwich.

"Is he as big as me, Carla?" Rocky asked.

"About the same, I guess. Could you get me a can of pop?" She looked up at me. "You better hurry, or you're gonna have to go." On cue, I came.

Carla didn't wait for me to move; she rolled off the bed and padded into the bathroom. "I gotta douche."

Rocky told me to tie up the end of my condom. I was still buckling up my pants as we crawled out the window. Carla came back into the room. "Hey, where's my pop?" she asked.

Sliding out the window, Rocky only answered, "Thanks, Carla, see you next week."

Outside, Rocky and I held our knotted rubbers up to the streetlight so we could, as Rocky put it, "compare loads."

We visited Carla regularly for several months, introducing more of our friends until a friend of a friend fell in love with her and made Carla stop seeing the rest of us.

Truth or Consequences

What did this kind of first intercourse experience do to David?

It set a very bad precedent. Women were to be used, and he felt he was to be in charge; he was supposed to be satisfied. He was supposed to do the work, and he didn't have to have any real feeling for her. David felt he could use sex to impress himself and his friends. It was easy and devoid of emotion, concern, or mutual respect. There were women to fuck and women to love, and it was hard to put the two ideas together. All his life, David struggled with intimacy, real intimacy in sex.

To this day, he still has a hard time sharing the control—not just because of his first intercourse experience, but because of the pattern it started, the groundwork it laid. Imagine what it did to Carla.

Some people might think that this wasn't such a bad or traumatic first intercourse experience. But it obviously put sex in the "selfish fun and ego boost" arena for the boys and "use me as a semen receptacle" for Carla.

I think it's a lot harder to learn to add love to sex than it is to add sex to love. If you start with sex, you risk never getting the two together, whereas starting with love and caring gives you a better chance of melding the two together as they should be.

9

Sexually Transmitted Diseases

There are over 35 sexually transmitted diseases out there. Gosh, they're getting to be as popular as ice cream flavors. Some STD flavors of the month: chlamydia chocolate, cherry gonorrhea.

> *Every 15 minutes someone dies of AIDS in the United States. Every 9 minutes someone is diagnosed with AIDS. Every 13 minutes someone is infected with HIV.*
>
> *Americans suffer more than 12 million cases of other sexually transmitted diseases every year. These STDs include gonorrhea, chlamydia, herpes, and hepatitis B. More than two-thirds are among young people under 25—and 3 million are among teenagers.*
>
> —Centers for Disease Control and Prevention. *HIV/AIDS Surveillance*. Atlanta: CDC, 1993.

I don't believe that the threat of catching an STD, even AIDS, is enough to change our sexual behavior. Fourteen years into the AIDS epidemic, researchers seem amazed that in some groups the percentage of people using condoms has increased only slightly or, in fact, decreased. I'm not surprised. The fear of pregnancy hasn't cut down on the incidence of vaginal intercourse without birth control. Fear doesn't change behavior for long, if at all.

If we were rational, the threat of a potentially lethal virus being transmitted into our bodies during anal, vaginal, or oral sex would deter us from playing sexual Russian roulette. But sexual expression is rarely rational. If we fear rejection, loneliness, or physical and/or emotional abuse more than we fear infection, then we cock the trigger, point, and squeeze. A series of empty chambers gives us the confidence we need to continue gambling. The fear of rejection can make us do loony things. We underestimate the pain of loneliness and the desperate desire to be needed, even for a superficial moment.

Sexually Transmitted Depression

Some STDs can be transmitted emotionally. A lot of us, myself included, have decided to have a sexual encounter with someone even though we didn't want to. We desperately needed an encounter, any encounter, even if only for one night or for five minutes. Almost unconsciously, we find ourselves performing the sex act. We pretend our way through it, even pretending to ourselves that it's great. We try to fill emotional needs with sexual acting out. But sex doesn't work this way. Instead it leaves us empty, hurt, confused, angry, and sometimes infected—just a little reminder of the experience.

Super Teen Denial

I often hear adults say that young people don't worry about STDs because they believe that nothing can possibly happen to them, but I don't remember feeling superhuman between the ages of twelve and twenty. I felt insecure. I fretted, obsessed, and cried about something every day. I worried a lot about death. I felt more pessimistic and fatalistic than at any other time in my life. I believed that I was a magnet for bad shit. And, I still took risks: I drove fast, drank too much, tried drugs, shoplifted, cheated, lied, broke rules, and ignored curfews. My need to try new things was much stronger than my fear of punishment. Whatever was most important to me at that moment took precedence over anything else. I knew I might get into trouble, big trouble, but I thought I would be in bigger trouble emotionally if I didn't go after what I thought I needed. I feared everything; one fear more or less didn't register.

I couldn't share most of my feelings. I knew that the world didn't like teenagers. Adults scarcely tolerated us. We were irresponsible pains in the ass, and they couldn't relate to us. They expected nothing from us. We resented our low status and made conscious efforts to live down to it. Some of us—head cheerleader, football captain, president of the student government—played the game better than others, but if *we* felt alienated, imagine how the nerds, druggies, and losers felt!

Like almost every other kid, I was wise to adults' habit of exaggerating the bad of something they didn't want us to do. We knew this tired old trick: it insulted our intelligence. It made us more anxious to rebel. Adults still use the same tactics: threats of hell and damnation and death. But threats don't work. Statistics say our chances of getting an STD are greater than ever, yet each generation starts having intercourse earlier.

We have better plumbing than our great-great grandparents. Modern medicine has found cures for syphilis and gonorrhea. We have better-fitting and more pleasure-sensitive condoms. We know how to track STDs and predict who will get them next, almost to the day, and in what situation and position. Meanwhile, another STD epidemic rages on.

You can catch HIV, syphilis, gonorrhea, venereal warts, chlamydia, and the whole gang of microorganisms and parasites from one sexual encounter, or you can luck out and have sex with a busful of strangers and catch nothing. But at this point I need to state the obvious: the more sexual partners you have, the greater your risk of taking home something you don't want. Our immune systems react to someone else's semen or vaginal fluid as alien substances. Our body's defense network works triple-time to neutralize those new invaders. Repeated assaults can leave it weakened. We weren't designed to overload our systems again and again with many different bacteria-filled fluids.

An immune system has only so much fight in it. Excessive stress can reduce the body's ability to defend itself. Drugs, including alcohol and tobacco, cause more destruction. Poor nutrition takes its toll, and pollutants finish off what's left of the body's defenses. A whacked-out immune system contributes greatly to the chances that a virus, once introduced, will grow and multiply.

Harsh Judgments Keep the Silence

Some people can laugh off an STD. They take their medication, then go out and catch a different one. Not many of us can shrug off a chancre growing on our genitals. Most people want to die of shame when they get an STD, which is precisely what keeps STDs spreading so fast. If I get one, I'm dirty, I'm bad, I've disappointed everyone I care about, my partner will hate me and leave me, I'm scarred for life, I am worthless. No one must know, I'll die of shame and embarrassment. The doctor's visit is humiliating, and depression sets in for months. Overwhelmed with shame like that, I can't tell my sex partner or partners I'm infected.

Whoever perpetuates the STD stigma does so as a deterrent, as if STDs separate the good people from the bad people. But judgments have never stopped an STD epidemic. They only promote fear and discrimination, because no one feels safe admitting that he or she has or has had a sexually transmitted disease. Silence takes over, denial sets in, and treatment often comes too late, causing others to become infected. Worst of all, those in need don't get the care and compassion that is their right.

Staying Cool While You're Hot!

Sexual judges don't tell the whole truth about sex and STDs. You can have sexual playtimes with yourself and others without risk of contracting an STD! You can have orgasms up the gazoo. You can feel great before, during and after, if you know how to be sexually cool when you're hot.

Most Common **Sexually Transmitted Diseases** *

STD	What is it?	What are the symptoms?	How do you treat it?	If you don't treat it?
Chlamydia	Bacterial infection spread through vaginal or anal intercourse or oral sex.	Most women and some men have no symptoms. Symptoms include discharge from penis or vagina, pain in lower abdomen, pain when you urinate.	Antibiotics from a doctor.	Can cause pelvic inflammatory disease in women and sterility in men. Can cause pneumonia and death in babies born from infected women.
Trichomoniasis (Vaginitis)	Parasitic infection which usually occurs in vagina in women and urethra in men.	Often no symptoms, especially in men. Symptoms for women are vaginal discharge, itching, burning or pain, and pain when you urinate.	Antibiotics from a doctor.	Symptoms will continue. May cause complications during pregnancy.
Gonorrhea	Bacterial infection spread through vaginal or anal intercourse or oral sex.	Discharge from penis or vagina, pain in lower abdomen, pain when you urinate or have bowel movement.	Antibiotics from a doctor, if diagnosed early.	Can cause pelvic inflammatory disease in women, sterility in men, skin disease, heart trouble, arthritis and blindness.

	How it is spread	Symptoms	Treatment	Complications
Syphilis	Bacterial infection spread through vaginal or anal intercourse or oral sex.	Painless reddish-brown sores on the genitals. About a month later, rash may appear, along with sore throat, fever, flu-like symptoms.	Penicillin from a doctor, but damage done to body organs cannot be reversed.	Can damage heart, brain, eyes, nervous system, bones and joints. Can result in blindness, heart disease and death.
Genital Warts (HPV)	Infection spread through vaginal or anal intercourse or oral sex.	Painless, fleshy warts on and inside the genitals, anus and throat.	Chemicals, freezing or laser therapy and surgery, but symptoms often reoccur.	Can cause cervical cancer.
Herpes	Infection spread through vaginal or anal intercourse or oral sex.	Often no symptoms, but blisters or painful open sores may appear on the genitals.	Antiviral drugs from a doctor, but herpes cannot be cured.	Can be passed on to baby during childbirth.
Hepatitis B	Infection spread through vaginal or anal intercourse, sharing drug needles, or piercing skin with contaminated instruments.	Often no symptoms, but flu-like symptoms may occur, such as fever, headache, fatigue, loss of appetite, vomiting, diarrhea.	Most infections clear up by themselves, vaccine is available.	Can lead to liver disease; can be passed on to baby during childbirth.
HIV	Infection present in semen, blood and vaginal juice. Spread through vaginal or anal intercourse or oral sex or sharing drug needles.	Flu-like symptoms that don't go away, weight loss, diarrhea, night sweats, swollen glands, white spots in mouth.	Symptoms can be treated by a doctor, but eventually HIV will develop into AIDS.	There is currently no cure for AIDS. Can be passed on to baby in the womb and in breastfeeding.

* We have put this chart together for this book, but we highly recommend that you order an even better chart called *STD Facts* from ETR Associates Network Publications, P.O. Box 1830, Santa Cruz, CA 95061-1830, 1-800-321-4407.

10

*S*afer Sex Is Better Sex

Long before HIV and AIDS came along, sex involved risk. Pregnancy and the long menu of STDs have always been dangerous possibilities. Now with new and better contraceptives, the recent availability of safe abortion, and the effectiveness of a shot of antibiotics in the old rear end, the danger has lessened. Even those embarrassing crabs that made you scratch your crotch like a baseball player can be washed down the shower drain with anticrab shampoo found in the same aisle as cures for jock itch, feminine itch, hemorrhoids, and athlete's foot.

When risks are lowered, however, so is fear. Our attitude toward genital infections becomes relaxed because if people know they can find an easy and confidential cure, they tend to worry less or not at all about prevention.

People frequently weigh the difficulty of avoiding risk in emotional as well as physical terms. If, for example, it feels emotionally easier for me to go to a clinic for a shot of antibiotics than to talk about condoms with my partner, then I'll risk infection. Likewise, if it feels emotionally riskier to go to a clinic and get fitted for birth control than it is to close my eyes and pray that I won't get pregnant, then I'll start praying and risk getting pregnant. For men, pregnancy is also a risk, at least emotionally. So is rejection. Men worry about ridicule if a condom slips out of their hand or doesn't roll down like it did on the practice cucumber. They live in fear of the worst scenario—the dreaded lost erection.

To Risk or Not to Risk

If it feels riskier to tell someone to stop pressuring me to try anal, vaginal, or oral sex than it does to just lie there and take it, then I'll lie still and risk hurt, guilt, and infection.

If it feels riskier to tell someone I've been raped, sexually assaulted, or harassed than it does to suffer in silence, then I'll risk lifelong emotional damage and be quiet.

Some of us may not understand why people risk their emotional or physical health to have sex, but risks are all relative and personal. Everyone has his or her own fears about sexuality, fears that may not be rational or based on common sense.

As destructive as these irrational fears can be, a false sense of security or a lack of fear can be just as dangerous. If, for example, a person takes a risk with anal intercourse and doesn't catch anything, the experience may induce a feeling of relief and power. Beating the odds—even just once—can fool a person into believing that the risk has been exaggerated. "I've had lots of sexual experiences, and I never caught an STD," they think. Then, when risky sex is connected to an STD epidemic like the current AIDS epidemic or an increase in unwanted pregnancy, those who were lucky can pretend that those who weren't must have done something wrong. They either deserved what they got, were members of a high-risk group, or were somehow different. Not true. Not smart.

The trick is to choose our fears and to identify risks carefully and rationally. We *should* fear STDs, because they're very real. We should take every precaution to prevent STDs—even though we may not catch one every time we have sex, and even though many STDs can be easily treated or even cured.

We should *not* fear saying no, being honest—or being rejected simply because we're being careful, saying no, or being honest. I promise you: having sex with someone you can't even be yourself with is *not* a risk worth taking.

The way I see it, the only thing you risk losing is a selfish, inconsiderate, unsympathetic partner.

Once Risky, Always Risky

Seeing risky sex in a historical perspective can make a difference. Today's dangerous sexual activities would have been just as risky a hundred years ago. There have always been fatal STDs. Though far fewer women face the risk of dying in childbirth today, for many the emotional trauma is as great as ever. When new cures are discovered, some generations get short reprieves from the risk of particular STDs. When just enough time has passed for everyone to feel really safe and free again, *wham!*—we're hit with a new "stronger-than-any-antibiotic" disease. HIV is today's special risk.

If we accept that some ways of having sex are eternally risky, then we're less likely to fall into the trap of false security. Above all, we've been using our genitalia all wrong, and that's the main reason why we keep getting into trouble. We could start using our genitalia correctly by reminding ourselves of facts that have been ignored or forgotten over the years.

Fact: All genitalia are germy, therefore genitals should be thoroughly cleaned with warm, soapy water before and after any form of sex. No exceptions. But soap doesn't kill *all* bacteria, and most antiseptics are too harsh for that area. Using your genitalia demands that you take precautions such as cleaning and covering to avoid nasty aftereffects.

Fact: Certain body parts aren't meant for certain sexual activities. You may break or damage them, and your parents can't buy you new ones! So everyone who intends to engage in sexual activity should learn the relative risks of their behavior.

If you use this part of your body for sex . . .	*Then these activities carry risks:*
Anus (butt)	*Most risky*: any contact with a penis not covered with a condom; inserting large, hard, sharp, unclean objects (bottles, wrenches, fil-o-faxes, etc.).
	A little less risky: contact with a penis using condoms (use two).
	Least risky: inserting fingers with short, smooth, clean fingernails.
Vulva (including vagina)	*Most risky*: (as above)
	A little less risky: contact with a penis covered with a latex condom with an additional method of birth control such as foam or gel spermicide and/or a diaphragm.

Least risky: fingers with
short, smooth, clean
fingernails; clean dildos
and vibrators

Mouth

Most risky: contact with a
penis not covered with a
condom, swallowing
semen; contact with a
vulva, swallowing
vaginal fluid; contact
with an anus.

A little less risky: contact
with a penis covered
with a condom; using a
latex barrier between
mouth and vulva, or
between mouth and butt.

Least risky: contact with
lips and tongue, clean
fingers and toes, breasts,
nipples, shoulders,
elbows, necks, stomachs,
thighs, etc.

Fact: Our bodies were not meant to handle bacteria-saturated semen and vaginal fluid from a lot of different people, or butt germs.

Fact: Lesions from STDs, such as syphilis and genital herpes, facilitate transmission of HIV. In one study, 38 percent of sexually active teens had the human papillomavirus (HPV), which causes genital warts and is associated with a higher risk of cervical cancer. Many STD infections are asymptomatic or display symptoms that adolescents do not recognize. Left untreated, STDs can result in death, pelvic inflammatory disease, ectopic pregnancy, infertility, neoplasia, adverse pregnancy outcome, infant pneumonia, infant death, mental retardation and immune deficiencies.

—Advocates for Youth (formerly The Center for Population Options), *Adolescents, HIV and Other Sexually Transmitted Diseases, The Facts.* May, 1993.

The Riskiest of Risky Sexual Activities

Anal intercourse (putting a penis in a rear end) has always been risky because of the way the anus is constructed, whether it's attached to a man or a woman. Its purpose is to excrete feces, the most germ-filled human waste product. The thin tissue inside the anus tears easily. Even an accidentally eaten nutshell passing through the anus can tear this delicate tissue. It doesn't open wide, either; being stretchy isn't its job. Poops are usually smaller and much softer than a penis, so putting a big, hard penis in there can cause damage, and even extremely tiny tears can be risky. Fingernails are dangerous, too. Anything used too vigorously will cause damage.

As the entire pelvic area becomes sexually aroused, the feeling of stimulation can spread to the anal area, too. Nothing wrong with that, but it can fool us into thinking that we can use the anus *the same way* we can use the vagina. Wrong. Every person's genitals have their strong and weak points, and the anus is not one of the strong ones. If there's a tear in the walls of the anus (and I'm talking microscopic here), bacteria, germs, and viruses (including HIV) can be deposited directly from a penis into the blood system. Even if there are no tears, some germs can still go through the tissue of the anus and can cause infection. Even dirt from fingernails can cause infection. HIV didn't make putting a penis in a rear end risky. Hemorrhoids, herpes, viral warts, gonorrhea, and syphilis have always been risks of anal intercourse.

Playing in this area takes finesse, caution, and complete knowledge of the risks. Putting any object in the anus is risky, even when done carefully. I know, many people like anal intercourse. But please, weigh the risks against the pleasure.

Reasons people give for having anal intercourse:	*Reasons why they should think twice:*
I can't get pregnant.	You can die.
It's the only penetration I can offer.	Try your hands, your mouth, your big pecs pushed together!
I want his penis and semen inside me.	You'll get his lethal microorganisms, too.
It feels good, so I can accept some risk.	It feels just as good with a condom; the anal passage doesn't feel the difference!
Technically I'm still a virgin.	*Now* I've heard every rationalization!

Silence Increases Danger

Don't say a word about anal intercourse. That's the attitude of most of society, which still regards it as a taboo subject. Some of us first hear about it through jokes or occasional discussions in an ominous tone with a snicker. We quickly realize that anal intercourse is a real no-no, and only dirty, perverse people would do it. "I mean, vaginal intercourse is gross enough, but *that* is unthinkable." By hiding the truth, we allow mistaken deductions that fuel fear, judgment, and ignorance to take hold.

"If this is done by perverted, gross people, then those people who do it must be bad people. All gay men must do it, because that's all they really can do. Therefore, gay men are perverted."

In fact, not all gay men try anal intercourse. But one out of four college women do. That means that a whole bunch of heterosexual men do it, too, because women can't do it to themselves. And think about this statistic: According to a *Redbook* magazine survey, 43% of married couples have tried it, for all sorts of reasons. Snickering definitely fuels the fascination. For some, the stigma attached to anal sex makes it even more attractive. And since we know how easily people lie about their sex lives, then even more people are probably trying anal intercourse and denying they do.

The aura of perversion surrounding anal sex keeps any honest information about it hidden. People can't follow safety precautions when they don't know about them. When taboos make the act itself unmentionable, no one can ask a pharmacist which condoms provide the most safety in anal intercourse.

Knowing and acknowledging why we want to participate in a sexual activity is as important as knowing the risks of that act. Someone wanting to put his penis into my rear end doesn't necessarily want *me*; it does mean that he wants my rear end for his pleasure. It also doesn't necessarily mean that he thinks I'm sexy or attractive; it only means that at this moment he believes my rear end is a good place to put his penis. Now, he could *also* love and want me. But if he and I both know that this is an extremely risky act, especially on my part, and he still presses me for my okay, then his definition of love is emotionally and physically risky for me! There are other forms of penetration without as much risk.

People can have anal penetration without harm using

gentle stimulation with fingers or soft, small sex toys. Sexual arousal will make the anal passage more receptive to penetration. Play carefully, or anal intercourse may end your playing forever!

Not all males who practice anal intercourse are homosexual or bisexual. There are some data that suggest that some bisexual men enjoy anal sex, but so do some heterosexual men. The Kinsey Institute reviewed seven studies and surveys conducted over the past 40 years to derive an estimate of the number of women who have experienced anal intercourse at least once. Our conservative estimate is that 39 percent—or more than one in three—have done so. In a recent Kinsey Institute study of college students at a Midwestern university, almost 24 percent of the women and 27 percent of the men reported having tried anal intercourse at least once.

—Reinisch, June M., Ph.D.,
The Kinsey Institute New Report on Sex. St. Martin's Press, New York. Page 137.

The Risks of Vaginal Sex

Vaginal intercourse has risks similar to anal intercourse. Plus someone could get pregnant. But the vagina was designed to accommodate a penis, and it is stronger and tougher than the anal passage. The tissue inside the vagina doesn't rip or tear as easily as anal tissue; it can take some thrusting, prodding, poking, and friction without being injured. It is certainly not indestructible. Don't let someone play "pile driver" with his penis or anything else.

Thrusting too hard and too long can cause irritation on the inside and back walls of the vagina, allowing germs, bacteria, and viruses to enter the bloodstream. The opening at the back of the vagina, the cervix, allows sperm and germs to enter the uterus and the bloodstream. Also, thrusting a penis in and out of the vagina can push against the urethra, from which a woman urinates, forcing germs into her bladder and causing urinary infections. And, of course, sperm can enter the cervix, creating pregnancy.

"But my vagina is made for use, isn't it?"

Yes, use—not abuse.

Play gently. Don't use a vagina as a punching bag or a place to put semen thoughtlessly. Use latex condoms correctly every single time a penis *touches* or enters the vagina, with additional effective birth control (see chapter 11). A woman should let her sex partner know that she expects him to pull out before orgasm. Now withdrawal is a problem in and of itself. It's never really worked for birth control, and now I bring it up for added HIV and STD protection. In this context, it is *added* protection to be used with the condom. From the "receiver's" perspective (i.e., the one with the penis in her or him), it's almost impossible to ensure that your partner will pull out, especially (and here's the catch) if you don't know and trust him. Obviously, if you don't trust this person well enough to pull out, you don't know him well enough to penetrate you! If your partner has proven to be caring and considerate in other areas of the relationship and at other times during sexual play, then this shouldn't be a big deal. If the person balks, whines, complains or refuses to pull out, then he doesn't deserve to be in there in the first place. A man should also be sensitive to changes of sensation during intercourse that can indicate when a condom has broken or fallen off.

It amazes me to hear stories about what women allow men to do to their vaginas. It's even sadder to me that another generation of young women has been brought up to believe that a man's pleasure is more important than a woman's life. Vaginal intercourse is, and always will be, a high-risk activity for women.

And you guys aren't out of the woods, I mean vagina, either. When a penis gets irritated from too much dry friction, germs can enter your blood system through small sores. The end of your penis has a hole that opens into two tubes, one for urine and one for semen. These tubes are made of delicate tissue that can also become damaged or irritated during vaginal intercourse. Add the risk of STDs and there's enough risk for you, too.

The Risks of Oral Sex

Finally, let's look at oral sex: putting a penis in your mouth, putting your mouth on a vulva, putting your tongue in a vagina or anus.

Putting a penis in your mouth puts you at risk of receiving STD germs. (It also may activate the gag reflex, which could possibly induce hurling!) If a guy has sexually transmitted bacteria or viruses on his penis, they can be transmitted to the mouth. Some germs on the penis skin or in the preorgasm fluids, as well as semen, are capable of going through the membranes of the mouth and getting into the blood system. And if the penis rubs too hard and long in the mouth, it can cause rubbing sores inside the mouth.

Something similar happens when a mouth comes in contact with a vulva and vagina. Vaginal fluid, like semen, is germy stuff that carries a risk. There is also an added factor: women can have blood (small amounts, usually) in their vaginas even when they are not having their periods, which means there is a risk of HIV infection when even a small cut or sore is present in the mouth. Sounds strange, but it's true.

Women sometimes bleed a little from their vaginas two weeks before (or possibly two weeks after) their periods. We don't always know why this bleeding occurs, but most of the time it's harmless. This does, however, add risk to the person performing the oral sex. (A woman who bleeds a lot aside from her period could have an STD. She should have this checked immediately.)

When oral sex involves the rear end, germs too numerous to count get introduced into the body via the mouth. And most people have some hair there, which catches nasty stuff that might cling while the rest gets washed away. Parasites that live in feces, if swallowed, can colonize in the digestive tract, causing pain and diarrhea, which is difficult to cure. Soap and hot water are good cleaners, but they cannot kill all germs.

Oral sex, especially oral-anal sex, is risky enough to use precautions and barriers. Couples want to know if they can ever have sex without the barriers and worry of risk. The answer is yes, if:

- Both partners have been tested for all STDs and have remained 100 percent faithful for at least one year after the tests were taken.
- Effective and reliable birth control is used correctly on a committed and consistent basis. No "I forgot to take my pills," or "I can't find my diaphragm."
- Each partner cares more about the other person's emotional and physical well-being than their own moment's pleasure.
- Sex toys like vibrators are kept clean and are not shared with friends or neighbors.
- You are committed to the idea that safer sex is real and better sex.

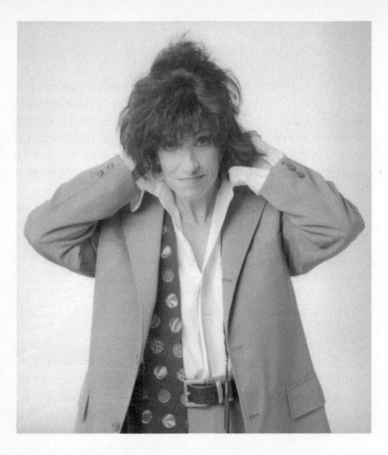

Promises of love break more often than condoms.

Condomania

Maybe Americans hate condoms because thinking about them undermines romantic myths about intercourse by reminding us of the consequences. In my opinion, that reminder is a plus.

Some statistics from the Centers for Disease Control and Prevention:

- Studies have shown that using latex condoms consistently (each act of intercourse) and correctly (from start to finish) does protect against HIV. Some people use studies of condoms as a birth control method to say they don't work. Comparing studies of condom use for birth control and condom use to prevent HIV transmission is comparing apples and oranges. Consistency of condom use is different, depending on the reason for use and other factors. For example, research shows that only 30-60% of men who say they use condoms for contraception actually use them every time. Even people who use them every time may not use them correctly.
- Studies of couples in which one person is infected with HIV and the other is not (known as "discordant couples") show that latex condoms are highly effective when they are used consistently and correctly. In

one study of 123 discordant couples who used condoms every time they had sex, *none* of the uninfected partners became infected. But among 122 couples who used condoms inconsistently, *12* uninfected partners became infected.

- Some people have said condoms frequently slip off or break, so they aren't effective. Studies have shown that condoms are not likely to slip off or break if used properly. In one study, only 1 condom out of 237 completely slipped off during sex and only 1 of 237 slipped off during withdrawal—1 of 237 is *0.4%*. In another study, breakage rates were less than or equal to only 2%. Every condom made in the United States is tested for defects and must meet strict quality-control guidelines enforced by the federal Food and Drug Administration (FDA).

- Others have claimed that condoms leak and don't stop viruses like HIV. But FDA conducts random tests of condoms using a "water test" to ensure they don't leak. Condoms are filled with 300 milliliters of water and checked for leaks. For condoms to be sold, 99.6% tested must pass the water-leak test.

- FDA has done further tests to find out if HIV can pass through microscopic holes in condoms or through the latex itself. They tested condoms with liquid containing tiny HIV-sized beads, at a concentration 100 million times higher than the concentration of HIV in people who are infected. They also tested using a live virus *smaller than HIV* at a concentration 10,000 times higher than HIV.

Even with the threat of HIV, not enough people use condoms. This surprises some experts, but not me. Sex educators thought that AIDS statistics would make people rush to pharmacies where they'd load up shopping baskets with rubbers. And if that didn't do it, then celebrities speaking out about having HIV would drive up condom sales. This never happened. Recently, annual sales actually dropped. Everyone from researchers to condom manufacturers and marketers have speculated on this phenomenon. They blamed:

- Their inability to advertise, specifically on television
- Uncertainty as to how to reach the people most at risk
- The religious right
- The public's embarrassment
- Fear tactics by AIDS educators that turn people off and push them deeper into denial
- A general lack of knowledge about condoms
- TV and movies, which don't include condom use in sex scenes

More people will start using condoms when attitudes change. Up to now, every ad that uses sex to sell a product has perpetuated the notion that great sex, specifically intercourse, is wordless and spontaneous. It's about time that advertisers started selling sex images that include condoms as well as the postponement of intercourse. I'd like to see condoms promoted as casually as seat belts and beer.

Finally we have an administration in Washington that promotes condom use through public service announcements on TV. But as of this writing, ordinary commercials for condoms still don't exist.

Campaigns that promote condom use for the most part have been targeted at men. But conquering men's resistance to using condoms hasn't happened, so the newest attempt has been to get women to demand that their partners use them. But before women can demand condom use each and every time, they have to feel the strength that comes with self-worth. (However, let's not assume that insisting on a condom is easier between two men. It's extremely difficult to demand behavior from anyone you fear or believe to be more valuable or powerful, whatever that person's gender.) A decade's worth of AIDS statistics can't counteract centuries of women's putting themselves second to men and their needs. As long as women believe that sex means more to men than to themselves, then men who don't feel like using condoms will get their way.

Of course, I understand that some men don't see that they use women. It wasn't until recently that the word *obey* was removed from most wedding vows. Women are entitled to have complete control over their lives and well-being, accepting no abuse and allowing no *use* without permission. If men have been unconscious up until now about their actions toward women, it's about time they became conscious. Putting on a condom may seem like a simple act, but this simple act can change history.

Many AIDS educators are now offering self-esteem courses for women. Cultures that have accepted sexist beliefs and laws for thousands of years can help defeat an individual woman's attempt to demand that her partner use a condom. In some households the risk a woman takes asking her mate to use a condom is more immediate than her having sex without it; *maybe* she'll get infected, but *for sure* she'll be beaten.

These little pouches of latex carry such symbolic meaning. They represent society's inability to deal openly with sexuality and with the reality of sexual penetration. Hand condoms out, and people will giggle, crack jokes, blow them up, and bat them around the room like beach balls. At my performances some people refuse to take them: "No thanks, I don't need one." Translation: "I'm not having sex—I'm a good, clean, moral person." Other people say, "Hey, give me a dozen for just tonight," or "Got any extra large?" Translation: "I'm Mr. Stud." When worn on someone's clothes, they symbolize an aggressive sexual coolness: "Yes, I have safer sex and am proud of it, so what?" When carried in a purse or wallet but never ever used, they symbolize intellectual support for safer sex but the fear to try it.

In the meantime, condoms are relegated to a corner of the pharmacy, usually by the prescription counter, so everyone can watch you pick out your favorite brand. To help change attitudes, and to make safer sex better sex, I cofounded a chain of condom stores called Condomania, where the selection of condoms is greater and there's always someone knowledgeable to show you how to use them correctly.

No matter where you buy them, no matter what shape, size, color, texture, or scent you use, just be sure to use condoms every single time you have anal, vaginal or oral intercourse (sex).

Correct Condom Use

[You have my permission to photocopy this whole section to give to a friend, lover, brother, sister, son, daughter, Mom, or Dad!]

Before you open the package, know that:

1. Only latex condoms stop the AIDS virus, not lambskin.
2. Condoms are effective only when used correctly.
3. You need to be aware of where you keep them. Don't store condoms in hot places (over 140°), in direct sunlight or freezing temperatures, or where they can get crushed or punctured. Avoid keeping them in your wallet (which a lot of men sit on all day) or loose in your purse (where sharp objects can put holes in them).
4. Condoms deteriorate with age. Check the expiration date on the box. Toss 'em if it's time, or if you believe a condom is over two years old.

Definition: Condoms can be made of latex or animal membrane, and soon plastic versions will be for sale. Lambskin condoms don't protect against HIV infection and they're less effective against other STDs. Condoms come in different colors; dry or lubricated; contoured or smooth or textured; and with slight variations in size.

Size: Condoms range in size from six inches to eight inches. Six-inch condoms are usually called snug fit; eight-inch are called names like Maxis and Magnum. Regular condoms are seven and one-half inches long. They always advertise the bigger ones in men's magazines—never the smaller ones. Who's zooming who?

Shape: Condoms come in two basic shapes:

1. Straight sided

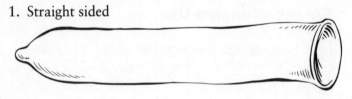

2. Contoured (shaped more like the "real" thing!)

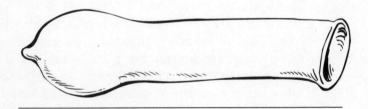

Fun Condom Facts

1. A condom can be stretched to the height of the average fourth-grader.
2. A condom can hold an average of 4 quarts of milk.

3. A condom can fit on the head of any player in the National Football League.

Not-So-Fun Facts About Condoms:

1. Among high school students who said they were sexually active, only 45% reported using a condom during their last sexual intercourse.
2. Most sexually active people are not using latex condoms every time they have sex. A national survey of heterosexual men with multiple sex partners found that only 17% used condoms all the time.
3. In another study, only about 20% of sexually active women reported that their male partners used condoms.
4. A San Francisco study of heterosexual men with multiple sex partners found that only 6% always used condoms.
5. A national survey by the Medical Research Institute of San Francisco, Berkeley, California, found that risky behavior is common. Of 2,058 adults (older than 18), 13% reported having had sex with more than one partner in the previous year. Most of those surveyed said they do not use condoms regularly. Of those with more than one partner, only 7% reported using condoms consistently.

Which Condom for Which Sexual Activity?

Use condoms during:

- anal intercourse: putting the penis in the rear end
- vaginal intercourse: putting the penis in the vagina
- oral sex: putting the penis in the mouth; putting a mouth or tongue on or in a vulva and vagina

Warning: A small percentage of people are allergic to latex. If itching or rash occurs, stop use and consult your doctor. Fortunately, condom stores carry hypoallergenic condoms.

Why It's Easy to Use Condoms for Each and Every Sexual Encounter

- You can buy condoms in lots of places: convenience stores, pharmacies, grocery stores, night clubs, condom stores, and even some condom vending machines.
- You don't need a prescription. That's good, because by the time the doctor called you back, you'd have lost the desire.
- They're inexpensive. But someday someone will make a 14k gold-edged condom for people who only like expensive things.
- Condoms are easy to put on.
- They help prevent pregnancy, AIDS, and other STDs.
- They cause no medical problems. Doctors and injury lawyers could go out of business.
- They may even help erections last longer.
- They encourage partners to talk about sex and keep the lights on!

Effectiveness: When used correctly (and *that* is the key), condoms are very effective in helping to prevent STD and

HIV infections and pregnancy. But they are not 100 percent effective. Studies report up to 98 percent effectiveness. When not used correctly, condom effectiveness rates are lower. The better quality the condom is, the more effective.

Step-by-Step:

1. Open the packet carefully. No teeth!
2. You hold in your hand one condom, rolled up. Don't unroll it yet. Make sure you know which way it rolls down; there is an inside and an outside. Nothing is more embarrassing than trying to unroll a condom that's inside out.
3. Place the condom directly on the head or top of the penis. Keep it straight and evenly placed, not tilted beret-style.
4. Pinch the top or nipplelike end of the condom—not Mr. Penis—to push the air out, because that's where the semen is going. (Some condoms don't have a nipple end, in which case just pinch with fingers, not fingernails, about a quarter-inch of the end.) This receptacled end will collect the semen. Without this end space, semen can be pushed out the top during ejaculation.
5. Some condom-using experts put a very small dab of water-based lubricant about the size of a pea on the *inside* of the condom before they roll it on. This can increase pleasure for the wearer, but too much lubricant can make the condom slip off.
6. Roll the condom along the penis using two hands. Four hands work even better. Make sure that the condom rolls all the way to the man's pubic hair. If you don't roll it all the way, it can slip off too easily.
7. Grab the condom-covered penis and squeeze the condom onto the penis for a tighter fit.

8. If you want, you can add some water-based lubricant. Dab some on the end of the condom and slide it along the sides.

9. As you enter and move within your partner, keep checking the base of the penis, making sure that the condom is staying put and not riding up or coming off.

10. *Men take note*: For added protection! Always, always, always pull out before orgasm. Immediately prior to orgasm, the penis is its largest, and the condom is most likely to break. Before you pull out, it's considerate to warn your partner, who also may be about to come! (I suppose that's when you get the most flattering size measurement, too, if you care to stop and admire.)

11. If the condom slips off or breaks, don't panic. Simply put your finger (gently) inside and pull it out. If you can't reach it easily, ask your partner to help. After all, that's what friends are for! Wash the penis before starting again.

12. If you do come in your partner, pull out immediately, before the penis gets too soft, holding onto the condom so it won't slip off inside your partner. Then, starting at the pubic hair and holding on to the rim, pull the condom off the penis, being careful not to spill any semen on your partner.

13. Wrap the used condom in a tissue or toilet paper, then throw it in a trash can—not down the toilet. It can clog the toilet, or worse, not flush down, floating there for your parents or guests to observe.

A Condom Glossary, or the ABCs of Condoms

Anal intercourse.   This is for experienced condom users only. Use two condoms—strong ones! No oil-based lube. Because of the tightness of the anal passage (butthole), there is more pressure put on the condom, so go slowly and carefully. Pull out *before* you come, so if the condom has ripped or broken, no semen will be deposited inside. Remember, both people are at risk if the condom breaks or leaks, because during anal intercourse, the anal tissue can tear easily, which causes bleeding. Blood is a high-risk means of transmission, along with semen.

Birth control.   Condoms are an effective means of birth control, too, but not 100 percent. When used correctly and carefully, they can be 97 to 98 percent effective. Use a spermicide, too, if you aren't allergic to it. Pull out before orgasm!

Condom.   The condom was developed by one Dr. Condom in the 1500's for King Charles II of England. Charles was a very horny kind of guy. His courtiers worried that he would catch a fatal STD, so they called in Dr. Condom to come up with protection for the king. Dr. Condom made the first condom out of sheep gut, doused in perfume and decorated with ribbons. In 1840 rubber was substituted for animal membrane, hence the nickname "rubbers."

Dental dam.   Not as big as the Hoover Dam. A dental dam is a square piece of latex used by dentists during oral work. The dentist places the latex square in the patient's mouth as a barrier. Same idea when used during oral sex. The dam is stretched across the vulva covering the vaginal opening and clitoris, allowing stimulation but no exchange of saliva and vaginal fluid. The dam is thick and tastes bad. Condom stores sell vegetable-dyed dams with flavorings, an improvement. A condom works just as well—just cut it up the side lengthwise and spread it out. Use dry, flavored condoms.

Erection.   You can't wear a condom without one! *Every erection* can be fitted with a condom. No erection is too big for a condom. Or too crooked. Or too fat. Or too small. If you lose your erection while putting on a condom, don't panic. Keep practicing. Practice at home by yourself. Have your partner stroke your penis while you put the condom on. If you like the way your erection looks, it will look just as good in a condom!

Fit.   Find a condom that fits. This means trying several different kinds. Not only should the condom fit the size and shape of the penis, it should also fit the sexual act. Lubed for anal and vaginal intercourse, dry for oral.

Gay.   To be happy! Everyone has the right to be happy about who they are and who they love. *Gay sex.* To be happy about who you share your physical, emotional, intellectual and spiritual being with.

HIV.   Before HIV, condoms were pretty much ignored by the general public. Even with other STDs rising at epidemic proportions, advertisers and the media were afraid to push for greater awareness. HIV made latex a reality. The word *condom* is easier to say now. Embarrassment subsides when fear increases. It's time for all of us to grow up sexually.

Inexpensive.   Condoms are anti-inflationary!

Kids.   Kids need to know about condoms. *Knowing* about something doesn't encourage use—it encourages more *knowledge*.

Lubrication.   When people are truly sexually aroused, natural lubrication flows. But stress, medication, and other physiological and psychological concerns can lessen or even stop this process. You may want to use a lubricant, never forgetting that when using a condom, only water-based lubrication will work. (Any oil—such as the mineral oil in moisturizers or petroleum jelly or butter—weakens latex in a matter of seconds.) Plenty of new lubricants on the market are sold in condom stores. Use them sparingly. You can also put a small dab on the inside of the condom before you roll it on to give extra sensation during play.

Masturbation.   Masturbate with a condom. Find out how much pressure a condom can take and which ones feel and fit the best. Be your own condom expert. Practice how to put them on and take them off easily without breaking or spilling the semen.

Nonoxynol 9.   This is a spermicide, a chemical that kills sperm and isn't harmful to latex. But a lot of men and women are allergic to it or get a bad reaction from it. Test yourself before using it. Get a foam or jelly spermicide and put it in the vagina before trying it during intercourse. If you get a burning or itching sensation, don't use it. Most lubricated condoms with nonoxynol 9 have a small amount of the spermicide and won't cause a reaction, but it's better to find out before the fact. Concentrated amounts can also affect the penis, causing a rash and blistering.

Oral sex.   Yes, it's risky! Not just for HIV, but other STDs, too. Use a dry condom. Some are flavored but don't have a sweetener, which may not appeal to you. Many of the flavored condoms are just sold for novelties and are not good quality. For use on women: cut the condom up the side and spread it out as a barrier (see Dental Dam).

Polyurethane.   Not for covering wood, but for covering a woody! The new female condom (and some male condoms) are now made of polyurethane. So far, testing shows quality and effectiveness equal to latex, and no allergic reaction.

Quality.   There are good condoms, great condoms, and bad condoms. Some companies care about manufacturing a good product, and some don't. There are several organizations in the U.S. that test condoms, including the Condom Resource Center in Oakland, California, Consumer Reports and University of California at Berkeley. You can find their reports at most libraries.

Risky.   Almost everything in life has some risk physically, emotionally, intellectually, or spiritually. Knowing the risk is always better than not knowing. Condoms *lower* risk. They do not eliminate all the risk. Using them correctly makes them more effective.

Sexually transmitted diseases.   There are over thirty-five STDs. They come and go with every new generation. STD epidemics are not new to civilization. Medications improve, but then so does the strength and complexity of the organisms. The body's immune system is overtaxed by pollution, stress, pesticides, junk food, alcohol and other drugs, and all the other daily bacteria, germs, and viruses. What makes us think our bodies can handle this constant bombardment of new sexual germs without being overwhelmed? Swapping semen and vaginal fluid assaults our immune systems. So it's silly to think that it is not a major problem and an unnecessary attack on the system that keeps us alive and healthy! (See chapter 9 for a list of the most common STDs.) And remember: latex condoms help protect against all STDs, including HIV.

Take your time. Put condoms on carefully. Take your time. Don't worry about losing your erection. Erections can't be lost—only postponed, decreased, diminished, put on hold, or delayed. They come back. Watch out for fingernails and rings. Take your time; you're worth it!

Under duress. If you're trying to or having intercourse under the covers, in the dark, with your eyes closed, you're not ready for any kind of intercourse. Besides, you can't put a condom on correctly under those circumstances. Put the lights on, come out from under the covers, and have your partner help!

Vulva. Now here's a great word that's not used enough. It's the whole outside area of the woman's genitals. It's the clitoris, labia (flaps of skin on either side), and the opening of the vagina (see diagram on page 24.) As far as condoms are concerned, the vulva needs protection as well as the vagina. Keep semen and another's vaginal fluid off the vulva and out of the vagina.

Women's condom. It is finally here and looks like a good idea: a polyurethane pouch for the vagina. It can break like male condoms, but it can't get lost inside the vagina. It is inserted like a diaphragm. For the women who have tested it so far, there have been no adverse reactions. It is a good solution for men and women who are allergic to latex. It may not affect the male's sensation and should not affect the female's sensation. The hard rubber ring at the opening can hurt when pushed against the woman's pubic bone. No condom is made for playing "pile driver."

XXX Large sizes. Yes, some men need bigger condoms for comfort *only*! Every condom is made flexible enough and large enough to fit not only over every penis, but also over a man's head! So, find the most comfortable condom for you. If you have a large penis, especially the head or glans, unroll the condom about an inch or two, and stretch it on like a cap, then roll it down.

Just Say Yes!   Condoms help lower risk, they are inexpensive, they are fairly easy to use (after practice), and our society is finally dealing with our condomphobia.

Zenith.   The pinnacle. The top. The highest point. The best place to be is the zenith of self-worth and self-confidence. Taking care of yourself and others is the zenith of a society. It's not an "either/or" situation, it's a "both." Take care of yourself and those you meet. Reach your zenith in all aspects of your life.

So now you know about condoms—but practice makes perfect. The best way for a man to learn about condom strength and sensation is to put a condom on and masturbate with it *before* he uses one with a partner. (If it breaks before orgasm, you have played a little too hard.) Try again to make sure you can have an orgasm without breaking the condom. Women need to know what a condom looks like, feels like, smells like, and tastes like before using one on a partner. Practice rolling it down household objects. (Not your cat.) Try different brands with different features, like ribbed, contoured shape, nonlubricated. Find a condom that fits you or your partner comfortably, stays on, and doesn't break during your style of sexual activity. By the way, nubs, bumps, and ribs don't add extra stimulation during vaginal intercourse. So save the "studs" for your jeans!

Congratulations, Condom Graduate! Here's your Condom Expert Certificate Card. Carry it with pride, knowing you have contributed to a safer world.

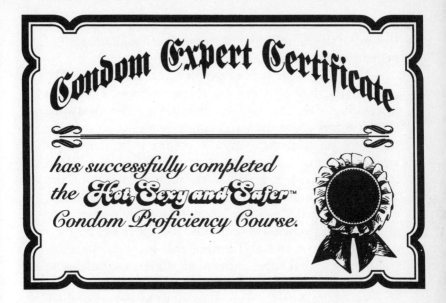

has successfully completed the *Hot, Sexy and Safer*™ Condom Proficiency Course.

The Condom Rebellion

I remember talking in history class about different rebellions, like the Boxer Rebellion. But I don't even remember what it was all about. I suppose today a boxer rebellion would be a great ad campaign in favor of "tightey-whitey" male underwear.

Men rebel so much more than women because men are encouraged to. Rebellion is part of developing into a man; it's a way to gain power and self-confidence. Unfortunately, sometimes too much power encourages entitlement rather than building self-confidence.

I say this because of the great Condom Rebellion of the 1990s. For over eleven years, AIDS and safer sex educators have been desperately trying to get men to use condoms for each and every experience of anal and vaginal intercourse.

Studies show that men are more resistant to condom use. Instead of this simple, logical, commonsense maneuver being embraced, a Condom Rebellion is still raging.

Not all men are part of the resistance movement. The great majority of gay men are using condoms. I find this fascinating from only one standpoint. Gay men deal with more penises (their own and someone else's) on average than straight men do. Now correct me if my analytical reasoning seems a bit askew, but wouldn't it seem more logical that gay men would be the most resistant and the most active condom rebels, since they are attracted to and celebrate the male "member" more than straight men? Not all gay men use condoms faithfully. Still, there has been no macho outcry or refusal. I assume that most gay men are still having sexual experiences of all different kinds, some that demand condoms and some that don't.

So why are straight men so slow to decorate their dicks? Maybe it's because straight men have been in the sexual driver's seat for so long that they aren't giving up the controls. Women, for as long as we've shared this planet, have been the ones to get, use and pay for birth control, even though it takes "two to make three." Not counting artificial insemination, of course.

The whole idea of the pleasure and need for sex has been male dominated forever. The "No one is going to tell me that I have to do something I don't want to do" sex syndrome. "I don't like condoms and I don't want to use one." Rebel yell: "I own my penis, not you! I'm in charge of my dick, and I'll use it when I want, where I want, and how I want." The fraternal pledge. This penis power has helped men maintain power and avoid being exploited. We rarely see penises on TV or in the movies unless they're xxx-rated. Women's breasts, buttocks and even crotches are freely shown all the time. How many *Playboy*-type magazines are there, compared to *Playgirl*-type magazines? Men are definitely in charge of their penises. I don't think it's embarrassment that stops them from being exploited like women's bodies, either. I think that they consciously or subconsciously know that if it is shown a lot, the power it has is diminished. It becomes a public object instead of a private part. Just the act of displaying it means it has lost some of its personal value and power.

So maybe this Condom Rebellion is about who gets control of the penis power. If the woman demands that a man wear a condom or there will be no intercourse, he has lost control over his own penis. Its beauty must be covered and hidden. The impressiveness of its magnitude and power is restricted, and then its potent juice is thrown away in a mini-garbage bag. Worst of all, its electrically charged nerve endings that produce the ultimate pleasure burst are diminished to one-half power, making the owner work harder for less reward.

The Condom Rebellion is alive and well, but there are a few traitors, and they are gaining momentum and strength. They have slipped over the front lines and joined forces with the "I can and still do have great sexual experiences using condoms" club. Club membership is rising. The quality and design of condoms are getting better. Condom-decorated dicks are a new fashion statement. This is a coed multicultural club with women wearing their own condoms and decorating their favorite penises with the best and most flattering latex wear. (A lot of men are dressed by their female partners and look better for it.)

Rebellions eventually end one way or the other. I think this one will end with most people becoming latex friendly, leaving only a few rebellious holdouts waving their unprotected penises around like flags, claiming their personal freedom rights. They probably don't wear seat belts either.

12

They Make Sex Look So Easy on Television

Sex on television looks so easy. Characters never forget to take off their shoes *before* they take off their pants. Nightgowns slide off effortlessly, drifting to the floor. And no one ever seems to smell anything unpleasant while making passionate love; no one farts or burps. They slip beneath the covers and dance as if under a blanket of clouds. They kiss slowly, melting to the ground or beach or bed or couch, catching themselves before they land. Cut to the moment after orgasm: they look perfect—no smudged makeup, bodies glistening with sweat.

We watch TV and movies with a strange idea of reality. We seem to know everything is make-believe, except the romance and sex. Even the apparent reality of sex in X-rated films is fake, fake, fake. Actors may have real erections and even real orgasms, but the seamless episode of endless sex you see consists of multiple takes, filmed over days and put together by a professional editor who tosses out all the stops and starts and whatever else wasn't in the script. And don't forget, actors never have to negotiate with the person they're in bed with about taking out the garbage.

American adolescents view nearly 14,000 instances of sexual material on television each year. Of these 14,000 sexual references on television, only 165 refer to topics such as sex education, sexually transmitted disease, birth control or abortion. This represents a ratio of about 1 to 85.

In all program categories, unmarried hetero-sexual couples engage in sexual intercourse from four to eight times more frequently than married men and women. Contraceptives are almost never referred to or used, but women seldom get pregnant; men and women rarely contract sexually transmitted diseases unless they are prostitutes or homosexuals.

Results from a study in 1987 found that after-noon soap operas contained 35 instances of sexual content per hour, or more than one instance every two minutes.

—Advocates for Youth (formerly The Center for Population Options), *Media and Adolescent Sexuality, The Facts.* August, 1991.

A Romance Thing or a Sex Thing?

I'd have been saved a lot of heartache, disappointment, and embarrassment if someone had told me that great sex and romance don't necessarily go together. Romance means tak-ing long looks into each other's eyes. Great sex, especially when intercourse is included, means taking long looks at what you're trying to do with which body part; one wrong move and someone could end up with an elbow in the gut.

Romance gives gifts like roses, gourmet foods, wine,

and even precious gems. Sex gives funny-looking rubber toys, fruit-flavored lubricants, and fluffy whipped spermicides. Romance wears sexy clothes made of satin, velvet, or lace. Sex wears latex—ribbed or smooth, powdered or lubricated, plain or colored, now *neon*! Romance moves bodies slowly in unison, to music, never missing a step and gracefully dipping to a reclining position. Sex moves bodies like tightrope walkers wearing combat boots during a tropical storm: badly aimed body parts, lost balance, kinks in your back, cramps in your leg, pinched breasts, trampled testicles, rattled bones and teeth, and sounds like those heard in a *Friday the 13th* movie. Faces can look romantic, but try to mimic your partner's face while he or she is having an orgasm, and see how romantic that is!

We do a real injustice to the inexperienced by telling them that great sex is romantic. Spontaneous romantic sexual interludes, more often than not, end up as disasters—emotional, physical, and spiritual disasters. Semiplanned, mutually satisfying, safer sexual experiences have a much greater chance of being successful and enjoyable to both partners.

Among adolescents, sexual activity is often unplanned and often occurs after drinking or drug use. One study of adolescents with unintended pregnancies found that almost one-half had been drinking and/or using drugs before the act of intercourse that resulted in the pregnancy.

The use of alcohol and drugs has been shown to inhibit the ability to practice safer sex or to use contraception at all. One study found that among sexually active adolescents who drink and/or use drugs, 16% used condoms less often after drinking and 25% fewer used condoms after drug use.

A survey of college students found that 75% of the males and at least 55% of the females involved in acquaintance rapes had been drinking or using drugs just prior to the attack.

—Advocates for Youth
(formerly The Center for
Population Options),
*Adolescent Substance Use and
Sexual Risk-taking Behavior,
The Facts.* July, 1991.

Lights, Camera . . . Do It

I've decided to take some lessons from Hollywood. First, I'm going to write the script with the help of my partner *before* a sexual encounter takes place. I'm going to talk about my ideas and expectations and find out what my partner envisions. Then we'll edit the script so that we're both happy with the story line. We'll codirect, passing the leadership back and forth, giving very clear, detailed instructions. We'll have lights and plenty of action. We'll discuss camera angles. We'll use as many takes as we want until we get the scene just the way we want it. We'll compliment each other's performance, and we'll never use stunt doubles. If either one of us finds the action too risky, we'll drop it from the script. We'll decide when the scene is over, making sure each of us is totally satisfied with our own work and our partner's work. And if it's Oscar material, we'll plan the sequel in the very near future! The best part is that the sexual encounter won't be a fantasy, we won't fake anything, and we'll get to cuddle with each other long after the scene ends.

Everyone who has ever been in a relationship knows that at first every phone call, every meal, every kiss seems romantic. After time passes and familiarity grows, romance dissipates; you wonder where it went and if it will ever come back. The good news about romance is that just like on television, it can be created and recreated. Get some props, the right lighting, costumes, a perfect setting, and you have romance. All you need is a willing partner and a romantic, positive attitude.

It's Only Pretend

The funny thing about fantasies is that they're often the opposite of real-life values, morals, sexual tastes, and attitudes. That's why they often freak us out. I pride myself in supporting the empowerment of women, and I don't fall for the image of women as passive sex toys and turn-ons. I'm sexually proud and confident and have created a sexually equal relationship, yet my fantasies are sometimes sexist, exploitative, and look more like an X-rated male-dominated porno flick. So, how does this happen? I would never do what I fantasize about. If I wanted to act out my fantasies, then they wouldn't be fantasies.

Where do these fantasies come from? There are probably several psychological explanations for this complex contradiction, but knowing why I have exploitative fantasies doesn't always make me feel okay about having them. So what should I do? Trying to get rid of my fantasies only makes them more bizarre and demanding. So I accept them. Sometimes I have exploitative fantasies: so what! They're only fantasies. I have no desire to act them out, and they don't have to mean anything other than that I have fantasies. I will see if I can change them, but I'm not going to obsess over this. There are so many more important things in my life that I need to work to change. Real things.

13

Getting Real on Daytime TV

A typical day in the nineties: Phil Donahue is arguing with parents, teenagers, and teachers about whether condoms should be handed out in schools. *USA Today* (and yesterday, and probably tomorrow) is still debating the need for sex education. And the college administrators where I've stopped on my Hot, Sexy and Safer tour are worried about the reaction of the trustees to an open discussion of sex!

But with all this chatter, no one on TV or in the newspapers ever argues about the important aspects of sex: comfort, pleasure, satisfaction. No one, neither Phil nor Oprah, asks the younger generation if they even like having intercourse. No one asks young women if they're having orgasms. As a society we'd rather keep debates on condoms and sex education going so we don't have to talk about real sex stuff. Instead of endlessly going back and forth about if it's proper to pass out condoms to young people, let's ask them if they're having intercourse in the dark, under the covers, with their eyes closed. If they are, they're probably much too embarrassed to put on a condom anyway.

What Good Is Sex?

Simply giving someone a condom won't make that person use it, nor will it make anyone want to have intercourse. End of story. Now how about if the talk shows dealt with some real topics: Why are we having anal and vaginal intercourse? And why are *fourteen-year-olds* "doing it"? Now here's a good Phil Donahue question: What do we use intercourse for? I've got some answers, Phil:

- To boost our egos
- To gain power over someone
- To achieve sexual satisfaction
- To feel accepted
- To express love
- To improve our self-images
- To impose guilt
- To avoid rejection
- To prove something
- To rebel
- To get affection
- To pay back an obligation
- To show sympathy (These are sometimes called "mercy fucks.")

Answering that question would really boost ratings. Next time I'm on a talk show, I'm going to open like this: "Even if I help to create a man's erection, am I responsible to fix it, and must I fix it through intercourse? No, Phil, that's his erection; he can fix it! Besides, how do I know that *I* created it; maybe he was thinking about someone else. Let her/him fix it. And if I am responsible to fix this one, who's responsible to fix the seven to nine erections he'll have throughout the night or that Big One pointing his way to the bathroom in the morning?" Now *these* are questions!

What is our collective attitude about intercourse? Maybe that's what we need to ask before we start passing out condoms. But we don't have time! Phil's hour is almost up.

You *Can* Say "Clitoris" on Daytime TV

Anything goes on daytime talk shows. If the Romans still fed Christians to lions, you can bet that daytime talk shows would bring their cameras. But not long ago when I informed the producer of one of these shows that I intended to use the correct term for a female sex organ, you'd have thought I was threatening to end TV as we know it.

After dozens of appearances on talk shows, I know the drill. The wet-behind-the-ears young woman/man who greets me and offers me coffee is called a segment producer. They'll give me an idea of what the producers want me to talk about. It's all set, they tell me. I'll chat with some celebrity teens about their sex lives, then take questions from the audience. I say I don't think that these TV teens will talk honestly about their sex lives, but they say not to worry, the host will help. I doubt it. The only help she could give would be to talk openly about her own sex life, and I don't expect that.

Ten minutes before airtime, I've been to Hair and Makeup, and now I'm being escorted by the segment producer (it's a woman) to the greenroom. Suddenly she disappears into a meeting. When she returns, she tells me that Standards and Practices (the censors) wants to know what words I'm going to use. *Penis. Vagina. Clitoris. Orgasm. Condom.* She disappears again. Two minutes later she's back, frowning.

"They said that you can say *penis, vagina, orgasm,* and *condom,* but not *clitoris.*"

Yeah, right. They think it's that easy to dismiss my

clitoris and that of every other woman! I say to the now-embarrassed segment producer, "Listen. If I can't say *clitoris*, I'm not going on the show." Five minutes to taping, and I add my reason in a quiet but firm tone: "I will not help to perpetuate the myth that our orgasms are in our vaginas." She doesn't move. I maintain a steady gaze.

She says, "I'll be right back."

Two minutes later, the executive producer is standing in front of me, flanked by my segment producer and a representative of Standards and Practices.

"Hi, I'm Nancy, the executive producer. Now, why is it so important for you to say *clitoris*?"

I patiently explain that by mentioning only the vagina I would support the mistaken idea that a woman's orgasm comes from putting a penis in her vagina. Don't expect me to pretend the most important private part of a woman doesn't exist. And don't ask me to promote the idea that the clitoris is unmentionable. Bottom line, I won't perpetuate the misconception that our orgasms are hanging out in our vaginas, waiting for a penis to come along and detonate us.

Now all three are staring at me. I tell them, "I can't go on without saying *clitoris*."

Without even looking at the Standards and Practices guy, Nancy says, "You can say *clitoris*." She smiles at me and walks away.

I must have said *clitoris* at least twenty times on that show, and every time I did, I noticed my segment producer looking at me happily from the wings.

We Need New Words for *Sex Education*

I think we ought to throw out the phrase *sex education*. We've already ruined it by fighting about who's going to do it and to whom they'll do it and how it should be done. We could use other phrases or ideas, like these: Everyone must obtain a sexual information license, along with your drivers license. Either that or a Sex Smart certificate, proving you are a certified Sex Smart Person. Or a Bachelor of Sexual Functions degree, or maybe even a Genital Registration Card validating that you know all about male and female genitals and how to use, not abuse, them or their owners . . . Just a thought.

Some Facts About Sex Education

On average, secondary schools offer only 6½ hours a year on sex education—fewer than 2 of those hours focus on contraception and the prevention of sexually transmitted diseases.

   —The Alan Guttmacher Institute, *Facts in Brief. Teenage Sexual and Reproductive Behavior.* July 15, 1993.

   In a 1991 Roper poll of 1,004 nationally representative adults, 94% said education is an effective way to help people avoid AIDS, and 80% said they were *not* tired of hearing about AIDS and the media has not blown the problem out of proportion. 82% said information for young people needs to be "pretty sexually explicit" to fully inform teenagers; 80% said information for adults should also be explicit. And adults clearly want help in talking about condoms with children—62% indicated that condom information would be very useful. Respondents also said they thought discussions on condoms should begin about the time children are 11 years old.

A 1992 study found that AIDS education and sex education resulted in fewer sex partners and reduced sexual activity. But it increased consistent condom use among those having sex.

A World Health Organization review of 19 studies of sex education programs found there was no evidence that sex education leads to earlier or increased sexual activity in young people—and, in fact, six studies showed that sex education programs actually lead to a delay or decrease in sexual activity. Ten of the studies showed that education programs increased safer sex practices among young people who were already sexually active.

—Centers for Disease Control and Prevention, *Fact Sheet: Condoms and Their Use in Preventing HIV Infection and Other STDs*. Atlanta: CDC, 1993.

14

*O*rgasm Stress

Some men worry about having an orgasm too quickly. And some women worry that they take too long to come. I don't know who set this sexual-satisfaction alarm clock. I refuse to follow rules that say sexual play ends just because one or both partners have an orgasm or say how fast or slow I'm supposed to orgasm!

I hate orgasm pressure. I hate being told how many I'm supposed to have and how I'm supposed to have them. The orgasm police have no place in my bedroom. If I don't have orgasms every time I have intercourse or sex that doesn't mean anything is wrong with me or with my partner. It's my choice. Besides, how I have orgasms may change as I get older and more self-confident. Worrying about orgasms only makes orgasms worrisome.

The Orgasm Convention

I heard about an orgasm conference in New Delhi, India. I'm not kidding! The international conference on The Orgasm. Big-time orgasm pressure, with delegates from around the world. One paper considered whether men can be multiorgasmic. I guess there's fear that women might be out-orgasming men. Now people can worry that they don't

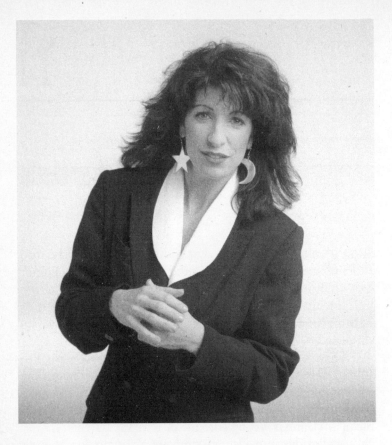

If you can't tell your partner what you want, how you want it, and where you want it, you're not ready to want it.

have enough orgasms and that the ones they do have aren't good enough. Orgasms ought to release stress, not add to it. I mean, if they're having this international conference at the same time the world is falling apart, then orgasms must be pretty damn important. True, they are—but maybe there's a happy middle place that would allow us to give out sexual information and encourage people to be orgasmic without putting so much pressure on them.

It might help to be aware of how we speak. Instead of "having an orgasm," I like the dynamic phrase "making an orgasm." Sounds artistic. Very hands-on, homemade, personalized. You could make one for yourself or for someone else.

No Hurry

Making orgasms is not something you should worry about or rush—that kind of pressure can ruin the whole process. Believing that you don't deserve one or that you don't look good during one can make orgasm almost impossible. I wonder if people who have trouble with orgasms are the same people who think that everyone looks good in that new style except them: "It looks great on her or him, but I'd look totally doofy."

Once (well, actually, more than once) I was having trouble making an orgasm with my partner. A counselor, he told me that I couldn't "let go," that I was afraid to give up control. That stressed me out even more. But after thinking about it, I realized that I had to agree. I knew I could make an orgasm by myself. I knew what I liked and how to do it. Our lovemaking just didn't include that stuff, and I didn't speak up and say what I wanted. Ideally, I could have showed him how and where to touch me, but I didn't want him to have control of my orgasm—or of me! I didn't feel close enough to him. I guess I just didn't feel safe in that relationship.

"I Needed That"

This past year I performed in a rural, working-class county way upstate in New York, at a community college. I love community colleges. Students come in all ages, with all sorts of life experience. With high school students attending that night, my audience ranged in age from fourteen to fifty-four! We had a great time. After the performance a woman, slight and short, came up to me through the crowd that was waiting for autographs and pictures. I almost didn't see her, but I heard her say something to me in a weak voice.

"Thank you so much, I needed to hear this. I thought . . ." Her voice started to break up like a cellular phone call. I put my arms around her and lowered my head to hear.

"I'm forty-five, and I've never had an orgasm," she sobbed as I led her to a corner. "I thought there was something wrong with me." I remembered my own confusion around how to have an orgasm during intercourse. She obviously didn't have a first love like Jim or a mom like mine. I could feel her tremble. The pain and tears weren't just about not having an orgasm. In her mind she wasn't a complete woman, she wasn't like everyone else. She was less— less sexy, less appealing, less valuable as a person and sex partner. The faking and pretending had worn her down. Her sexual failure was connected to all her other failures, and she couldn't find a way out. She was sure she couldn't tell anyone. Finally, another woman spoke for her when I appeared on stage and explained that my orgasm is not in my vagina, that intercourse by itself doesn't work for me, and that for most women, this is our sexual truth and reality: there is nothing wrong with us.

I'll never forget her face when she looked at me and smiled. "Take care of yourself," I said. She knew what I meant.

15

My First Orgasm

In the early sixties, Jude and I were the best in our sopho-more gym class, the most athletic and the most competitive. We were fifteen years old and great friends. The election of John F. Kennedy had released a mania for physical fitness across the country. In gym classes kids took fitness tests to measure themselves against national standards. We did hundreds of sit-ups, push-ups, and dashes as teachers stood by with clipboards rating our performances. The hardest one—climbing the rope—was the last test. This thick, knotted rope was hanging in the middle of the gym. To win this contest a kid had to climb all the way up to the steel girder where it was attached, touch the girder with one hand, and climb down in the shortest amount of time. No one in the class had made it past the first three knots. The rope was twenty feet high, but for most of the class it might as well have been twenty stories.

Jude and I were the last to try. We had gone through all the other tests, challenging each other all the way. The rest of the class watched, cheering us on like two gladiators. Jude went first, up the rope past the three knots. She was taller and thinner than I was, and she was fast. Clinging to the rope with hands and thighs, she inched her way up like milk being sucked up a straw. She banged the steel girder for effect, making a loud clang, and shimmied down the rope. Her time beat the national average by far.

A Girl and Her Rope

It was my turn, and I was ready. I loved adding this new adventure to a list of climbing accomplishments. I could do trees, monkey bars, rocks, porches, fences, and gymnastic equipment. A rope would be easy. I grabbed it and hopped on like a baby monkey, wrapping my thighs, strong from years of dance, around the coarse, hairy coil. I found I could pull my body weight with my hands and arms, but to stay on, my inner thighs had to clamp that rope like a vise. As I pulled and squeezed my way up the rope, it became embedded in my crotch. About halfway up, I started to feel funny. My body was becoming too tense. I was breathing too heavily for the amount of effort I was making. I didn't feel tired, just tense, but I was slowing down, so I pulled and squeezed even harder. I heard people saying, "What's wrong with her? Is she having a heart attack or something?"

The more I squeezed and pulled, the worse it got. I was panting for air and sweating all over. By this time, the gym teacher knew something was wrong. I was almost at the girder, but my muscles were so tense that I wasn't sure if I could let go to touch the beam. I heard her tell Jude to go up to get me. No way! I was determined to reach the girder. I was only inches away from touching it, so I gave one final yank, dragging the rope through my already-rubbed-silly crotch, and *wow*!—I started to shake and twitch, and the sweat poured out of me. My teeth clenched, and in ten seconds, it was over. All my muscles relaxed at once—a totally involuntary act.

Unsafe Sex

For a second I enjoyed the relaxation, until I remembered I was twenty feet in the air, clinging to a rope. I felt myself starting to let go and realized I could fall that way. It took the last minuscule milliliter of strength I had to force my exhausted hands and thighs to hold on as I slid down. Jude climbed back up to help me. She was halfway up when I hit her, knocking her to the mat on the gym floor. I landed on my back next to her. Gasping for breath, I looked up to see the gym teacher and the entire class leaning over me, screaming, "Are you okay?" I didn't know. I couldn't move. I was exhausted but relaxed. My hands and inner thighs were hot and stinging from sliding down the rope too fast—they'd warned us about rope burns—and the gym teacher wanted to send me to the nurse's office, but strangely, I felt fine. Just confused. What had happened to me? Jude was fine, but she had no clue about what had happened to me, either.

It was six months later, maybe more, when I discovered the answer to the rope mystery. My boyfriend, Jimmy, and I were horizontal in the front seat of his mother's car, face to face, with all our clothes on, and I was on top. We were kissing while our bodies rubbed against each other. I felt his erection against my lower abdomen. I inched up until it touched my pelvic bone and the soft flesh just below it. I didn't even have to spread my legs a lot. I could just move slowly, pressing his hard penis against my crotch. It felt unbelievable. I controlled my movements so that it hit that spot—the spot with all the pleasure. The more I rubbed, the better it felt. All my muscles tensed. I was breathing heavier, and I had a moment of déjà vu in which I knew I'd felt this before. We rubbed until I felt a burst of spasms radiate from my crotch throughout my whole body. This pleasure bounced around my genitals like a pinball being launched from bumper to bumper to flipper.

Eureka!

As quickly as it came on, the feeling subsided. I felt *sooo* relaxed, and just let all my weight lie on his body. As I lay there with this silly, contented smirk on my face, it hit me: that's it—that's what had happened to me on the rope. I began to laugh so hard that my boyfriend sat up and asked me what was wrong. I was laughing too hard to tell him, but I assured him that it wasn't him or what we were doing. He accepted my explanation reluctantly, and we drove home. I thought, *I hope it's not too late to call Jude.*

16

*G*ay, Straight, Bi, and Other?

I've had a same-sex experience. Actually, several experiences. But don't call me gay. And don't call me a lesbian. Or bisexual. Or heterosexual, either. None of those labels feel right to me. They don't describe me and my sex life. I don't go in for rigid definitions that confine us. Even people who accept these labels don't agree on what they mean. So count me out.

As far as I'm concerned, the following terms denote attraction to a gender—not necessarily who has sex with whom:

gay = a man who is attracted to and has sex with other men

lesbian = a woman who is attracted to and has sex with other women

heterosexual = anyone who is attracted to and has sex with the opposite gender

bisexual = anyone who is attracted to and has sex with both genders (not necessarily at the same time)

Most gays and lesbians have had heterosexual experiences, and many heterosexuals have had homosexual ones.
But attraction and identification means more to most sex
labels than sexual acts. Many people aren't exclusively anything, regardless of a label. Nor does their label mean that
they have anything else in common with other people who
wear their label, except sexual orientation.

People, Not Labels

Frequently labels convey much information. In my case, a
label won't tell you squat. Society wants to label me heterosexual because I'm having sex with a man. Because of my
sexual experiences with several women during my lifetime,
some will call me bisexual. But that label doesn't fit me,
either. I don't have sex with a woman just because she's a
woman. I am attracted to a whole person: attitudes, values,
talents, wisdom, sense of humor. Then I deal with gender
and genitalia.

After learning how to satisfy myself sexually, I realized
that I would probably enjoy touching and having a sexual
experience with a woman if I was attracted to her as a
person. Even though I was open to same-sex experiences,
my standards for beginning a relationship didn't change. I
still needed to love this person, trust her, respect her, have
important values in common, and want to work toward a
committed relationship. She had to be my friend as well as
my lover. It seems, at least for me, that the major difference
between a same-sex relationship and an opposite-sex relationship is the genitalia.

A lot of myths and stereotypes are still attached to
sexual labels, especially the bisexual one. That's probably
why I don't like it. Many people think that bisexuals have
sex for sex's sake. Bisexual people are characterized as
oversexed, promiscuous, and uncommitted to their main

partner. If you can go both ways, bisexual myth #1 goes, you'll have so many opportunities that you won't be able to control yourself. I'm amazed at these long-held misconceptions, but I understand why they attract believers. Most people who have had a same-sex experience never ever tell anyone. They don't talk about the sex, and they don't talk about the strong emotions such an experience can bring up. The bisexuals who do make the rounds on the talk show circuit don't speak for the millions of others who choose to remain private. I've never related to talk show guests who hold up their sex lives as if they were trophies.

We Are What We Are

In our desire to understand sexuality, especially the most provocative kind, we often try to make labels fit. We want to define groups by one sexual fact so we can reduce everything and everyone to simple common denominators. But people can't be defined that easily. Almost all of us are exceptions to the rule. Our quest is for greater understanding, but using labels only makes understanding more difficult; it also increases the amount of myths, misconceptions, and stereotypes we all have to live with.

Sometimes labels can help. Identifying with a group—social, ethnic, racial, gender, professional, religious, or almost anything—can encourage feelings of unity, loyalty, self-esteem, pride, and enthusiasm. Phrases like *gay pride* and *black pride* can promote healthy changes of attitude. Those born into groups that already hold social, economic, and political power are less likely to use slogans, because a sense of self-worth comes with the label. (White Anglo-Saxon pride? Christian pride?) But for others, there *is* strength in numbers and identification.

Just be careful about labeling yourself and others, because when labels hinder, they do so in a big way. Labels are almost always more restricting than expanding. They are society's shorthand, and shorthand doesn't give a full or personal picture. No abbreviation used to describe a human being will ever explain the person. My sex life can't be defined by one-word labels like *gay, straight,* or *bi.* When I talk about having sex with a woman, I prefer "same-sex experience." A same-sex experience doesn't come with a preordained lifestyle attached. Two people of the same gender had a sexual experience. Period. We don't know anything else about these 2 people—not their intelligence, humanity, or values.

Pride 1, Regrets 0

Writing this chapter was hard. I haven't told a lot of people about my same-sex experiences, because I worried about what certain people might think. Now, it seems almost chic. Not a good reason to do anything because it's stylish. I suppose I still haven't revealed much other than that I have had these experiences. I remember them with pride and no regrets; the women I loved are wonderful people: bright, loving, accomplished, caring members of society. I fell in love with them because of who they were as people, not what gender they were.

I smile when someone says that a same-sex experience is not real sex. Obviously, they have never had one. I'm not advocating a same-sex experience or relationship for everyone. I'm offering my experience here to clear up a few misconceptions and encourage tolerance. Tolerance doesn't ask anyone to agree with someone else's choices; it simply creates space for coexistence. It allows knowledge to replace ignorance and respect for individuals to replace hatred of groups. I do not lust after women because of my same-sex experiences; I do not leer at them in the locker room. If anything, I appreciate and admire women more.

Because of my experiences, I learned to love myself more as a woman.

Those who judge another person's sexual orientation probably stopped reading this book back at the table of contents. There are millions more who want to understand their own sexual experiences better, and if sharing mine helps, I'm glad. Everyone has the right to be proud of their sexual orientation. Everyone has the right to a sex life free of harassment and judgment.

Double Your Pleasure

Why do so many women get so scared and uncomfortable with the idea of two women loving each other and sexually expressing this love? Maybe because we as a gender are persuaded as little girls to hate our own "pee-pee." Hence: If my vulva is gross, touching another woman's must be even grosser!

But a lot of us don't really like men's pee-pees all that much, either. I mean, you don't hear a lot of women proclaiming the need to put a dick in their mouth. The thought of swallowing semen makes most women's gag reflex erupt like Mount St. Helens. Fondling a testicle can feel like playing with a cat's hair ball. Putting a penis in our vagina before we're ready is like wearing up-the-butt underwear on a hemorrhoid flare-up day. So why the revulsion and fear of lesbianism? I had a more commonsense approach to women loving women: If I like touching my female body I could probably enjoy touching another woman's body.

For many lesbians, but not all, being attracted to women means that they truly love and admire women. They believe in them and know them to be competent and strong people. And even in this homophobic society, women loving women doesn't seem to bother most men. This seems a bit hypocritical to me. Many times the men that want so much to see or experience two women together are the same men who violently object to two men having sex together.

It's a strange phenomenon that though so many women are attacked by men, a lot of straight women fear lesbians more. I've had female friends who have experienced male violence worry that a lesbian might attack them. My lesbian friends Trudy, Diane, and Sherry have had a lot of female lovers, and none of them have ever been attacked or sexually abused by another woman. Yet most of my straight friends have experienced violence from a man. Unwarranted fear based on judgment and myth only leaves us vulnerable to the real dangers.

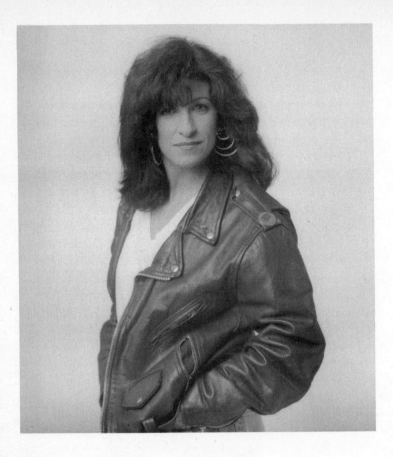

Show and tell is hot. *Do and brag is* cold.

17

The Best Turn-on: Honesty and Trust

The safer sex experts all say, "Communicate with your partner—discuss your sexual history. Talk about other risky activities, like IV drug use." Oh, sure. When we go into seduction mode with someone new, few of us will spontaneously bring up incidents of unprotected sex or the wanton exchange of body fluids. Most of us won't communicate the truth about ourselves until we know we won't get rejected. A simpler safer sex rule would read like this: "Don't have intercourse with someone until you feel safe enough to tell that person the whole truth about yourself."

At the beginning of a relationship everyone says what they think is necessary to make a good impression. "Oh, I'll eat anything. Shopping? I love it! Boxing? One of my favorite sports!" We accept this blatantly dishonest communication in order to continue the seduction.

The Anchovy Factor

The Scenario: The relationship is only weeks old, and the love lies have piled up.

SHE: Let's see, I've lied about liking anchovies. I've suffered through three Arnold Schwarzenegger films and complimented two tacky T-shirts, one ugly pair of pants, and a really bad new haircut.

HE: I should never have said I liked that perfume. It's on everything she touches. Why did I make such a big deal about liking her friends? I'll never stay awake through another double date.

BOTH: I'm so glad I said I haven't had sex with a lot of people, since he/she told me the same thing.

When couples who don't know each other end up in bed for a one-night stand, their minds race, but they're usually afraid to speak. I can reveal what goes on inside the heads of a couple like this:

THE FEMALE: He's got his elbow on my hair. Why does this always happen to me? God, is he heavy. He's rubbing my back trying to be sexy, but he really wants to find my bra hook. It's in the front! I wish he wouldn't suck on my bottom lip like that! This must be what it's like to make love to a vacuum cleaner. Now what? He's lifting my leg . . . *up over my head*. No way. Maybe he'd be happier with something plastic and inflatable. I'll just move him where I want him. Shit, I broke a nail. Okay, he's down there now; hopefully, he'll find it . . .

　　(Twenty minutes later.) He hasn't found a damn thing. Well, I can't be lying around here all night; I have a chicken defrosting at home. I know, I'll start the moan-and-groan bit, he'll think I'm getting excited, then he'll get excited, and we can move on to, "You're nice. Tell me your name again." *Ah, oh, hmmm.* Still nothing. Okay, this time I'll sound more like *The Exorcist* and maybe he'll get the idea.

THE MALE: Should I move her to the left? There. I guess she can tell she's in bed with someone who lettered in wrestling three years in a row . . . Oh, let's see if her leg goes over her head. Yikes! I got a fingernail in the back. I hate those things. Wow, she seems to be moving me all the way down here! I know what to do now: I'm a trained professional, ma'am, you just relax. I'll just, ah . . . or maybe I'll . . . shit, I wish I had a manual. I wish she'd speak up. Oh great, Ralphie decided to go lie down. I'll just look at her naked body—that'll get it back. But it's too dark. Okay, I'll ask her to light a candle . . . What's her *name*! Never mind, I'll just think of someone who always does it for me. Joey's girl-friend! . . . Oh good, Ralphie's happy. Hey, she touched me! Yeah, keep doing that, it feels great. No one ever did that to me before. Actually, it feels a little too good, and if she keeps doing it, I'm going to go too soon and feel like a jerk . . . I'd better think of something else quick, something to slow it down. Something unpleasant—my cat died today. Yes, think of DEAD CATS, DEAD CATS, SQUASHED all over the highway! *Aaahh!*

Note: Similar scenarios also happen with same-sex couples.

Hard to Be Honest

Even couples who live together for years in monogamous relationships have trouble communicating honestly. Those who meet and go to bed have almost no chance of telling or hearing the truth, no matter what their sexual orientation, race, or religion is. Almost all of us find it hard to communicate honestly. And being honest later in a relationship is more difficult if you weren't honest at the beginning.

Those little lies we justify in our relationship: "love

lies." A classic oxymoron, like "jumbo shrimp." No one I know has ever felt good about telling a love lie. And no one likes getting them. A love lie is supposed to spare a person from hurt feelings. In fact, our feelings are more hurt when we find out someone has lied to us. I've always had difficulty trusting someone's love anyway, so if someone I love lies to me, even about an insignificant thing, it weakens the trust I feel. I am the child of two alcoholic parents. (My mom was a recovering success story.) That made it hard for me to trust anyone. I learned to lie because I was afraid of my abusive dad. During his alcoholic rages, I lied to survive. We may justify love lies for good reasons, but they only hurt the chances of survival of the relationship.

My ability to trust grows the more I learn how to tell the truth. The more honest I am, the more I believe others are being honest. And even if sometimes they aren't, at least I know that I told the truth, and that makes me trust myself more—a necessity for self-confidence. You'll find other benefits to telling the truth: you don't have to eat anchovies, and you don't have to sit through three movies in a row that you don't like.

Origins of Distrust

Many people in couples don't trust their partners to be faithful. Their reasons are simple: "I've had someone cheat on me before," or "I've cheated and I know how easy it is to do." I think the problem starts earlier. It seems to me that the belief you can trust someone else and be trustworthy yourself begins the day you're born.

An inconsistent parent prevents his or her child from developing trust. "If my *own* mom or dad doesn't care for me—if they would rather drink, do drugs, use me as a punching bag, or sexually abuse me—who *can* I trust to love and care for me?" Unfortunately the relationship a child has with a parent often gets recreated later in life.

The paradox is that people who tell you they find it hard to trust are the ones who jump all too often under the sheets with someone they've just met. Say we meet in a bar, or at a club or party. We both drink until we have a good buzz on, each of us spouting total alcoholic bullshit. We go home together. We start fooling around. I don't want to have intercourse, but I don't say that. We have most of our clothes off. He thinks that I want to have intercourse, because I haven't said that I don't. In fact, we haven't said two words since we got here. I weakly object. He thinks I'm trying to pretend I'm not easy. I let the penis get close to my vagina. I say no. He pushes it into me. I think it's my fault— I went this far, so I guess I'm responsible. He feels and thinks he's entitled to my vagina, and if I didn't want this in the first place, why did I go home with him and why did I go so far? I thought I could trust him. He feels confused, angry, and misled. I think, *But he seemed so nice in the bar*. He thinks, *But she seemed so open and willing*.

I Like Noodles, You Like Noodles

Four hours spent getting bombed with someone does not create the basis of an honest, trusting relationship. The only thing you'll have in common the next day is a headache. Drunk or sober, we find the most trivial reasons to justify trusting someone we want to have sex with: we both like zipper jackets, sesame noodles, Chopin, ponytails, tall people, ice fishing, Buddhism, silent movies, Fords, kittens, bottled water. Having one, two, or even three things in common does not mean you can trust some half-stoned man or woman who has a nice haircut. Loneliness makes for a desperate need to trust too soon. We encourage each other to trust words instead of actions. We don't want to earn trust. And if we give it quickly, freely, no questions asked, and that person doesn't live up to our trust, we are crushed. We take no responsibility for our own overzealous trusting.

I know about this because I hold the Olympic record for being overly trusting. I still trust easily, but I've stopped trusting recklessly. I am aware of the human need to impress and to be liked, loved, accepted, and validated as much and as quickly as possible. Now I know that on the first, second, third, tenth, and twentieth meetings I don't always get an accurate 3-D image of the person I'm relating to.

And now I also understand the trust equation that so often blows up in our faces: We give lots of trust to someone we just met, a person who feels too insecure to tell us the truth. As this person feels safer because of our trust, they begin to tell us more truth. Then, when they finally tell us the whole truth, we don't trust them anymore!

Talk Is Cheap

Trust takes time. Sober time. And more than four hours of it. Enough time for actions to have more impact than words. Give yourself and your partner an opportunity to build trust one block of truth at a time.

Some people aren't to be trusted. They know it. We know it. Yet we allow them to talk us out of our feelings of mistrust because we don't trust our own intuition. We don't trust that we can make it without this dishonest person. We don't trust that we deserve better and can get it. We don't trust our ability to build a better relationship.

Great safer sex takes a lot of trust. Great mutually satisfying sexual experiences require a lot of trust. Sexual experiences that make you feel better physically, emotionally, intellectually, and spiritually are built on trust.

Safer Sex Means Never Having to Fake Anything

You know, it takes a lot of energy, mental and physical, to fake an orgasm. And don't tell me just women do it, because men can fake orgasms, too. They can't fake erections, but they can fake orgasms. So months, even years after the first fake orgasm, there we are, moaning, groaning, and writhing on cue.

But one night our partner notices. "Boy, it didn't take you long."

"I was tired—I mean, excited."

Then comes the first major argument.

"And you've never satisfied me. I just faked it."

Then, when you are making up: "Did you really fake it?"

"Of course not, honey. I just said that. You always satisfy me."

Faking any kind of sexual pleasure weakens the relationship the same way *love lies* do. I'd rather take all the energy I'm using to fake something and put it into teaching my partner what I like. If I'm too embarrassed to teach him or her, then maybe I'm not ready to do whatever it is I'm pretending to do!

18

*S*exually Act Your Age and Enjoy It

Grownups always said, "Don't have sex until you're an adult." They meant, *No intercourse for you, kid, until you're much, much older*. Some adults were just antisex. They meant *don't kiss, don't rub, don't touch each other's private parts even through your clothes, don't have an orgasm together*. I wasn't buying it. I felt my hormones kick in as a teenager, so I couldn't see postponing all sex almost *forever*. Anyway, I knew the word *sex* included a lot of different things, not just intercourse. Out of embarrassment, adults never seemed to talk clearly.

Our age and our sexuality always seem to be at odds with each other. Either we're too old for making out in the backseat or too young to have intercourse. People still say to me, "Act your age!" What the heck does that mean? I guess there's a chart somewhere—one I haven't seen yet—that specifies what you're supposed to do and when you should do it.

Now I'm an adult, and I have a different sensibility about sex and readiness: certain forms of sexual expression belong to certain times of your life. Some require a lot of communication between partners, some require more learned skills, some require comfortable locations that may not be available to the couple involved, and some require information that can be hard to find.

As with most things that require skill, one should master the beginner's levels before moving to intermediate or advanced levels. The process of learning new forms of sexual expression resembles that of learning anything new.

Tips for Beginners (those new to sex and those with new sex partners)

1. Don't start on the expert level. For example, hand holding is fine for beginners. Intercourse on a trapeze should be attempted only by experts. Holding someone's hand doesn't require you to bare your soul to another. Get the dirt out from under your nails and you're ready. It's the perfect expression for the inexperienced or newly acquainted couple. And talk about safe! No fatalities have ever been linked to hand holding. As I've already said, intercourse is the easiest sexual act to do badly and the hardest sexual act to do well. It takes highly developed physical, emotional, and spiritual skills.

2. Know all about your equipment and how to use it yourself *before* you let someone else use it. If you can't look at and touch your own body, don't let anyone else look or touch.

3. Keep your equipment in tip-top working order—have it checked regularly, and protect it from unfriendly elements and people who don't treat it with respect. Home care requires only soap and water. When the doctor takes a deep look, join in and see yourself for yourself!

4. Before moving on to a new level, make sure you've mastered the level you're at and that there's nothing you've overlooked. For example, beginners can practice rubbing and touching. This includes rubbing the whole body with your clothes on. Touching

your partner's genitals through his or her clothing offers a good introduction to someone else's private parts. It can also be extremely pleasurable and a form of *real* sex. Kissing on the cheek is a beginner-level activity. Somewhat more advanced activities include closed mouth kissing on the lips; open mouth kissing on the lips; kissing on the face, neck, ears, and any areas from the neck up. Ask your partner if he or she is ready to move on to the next level—kissing below the neck. Sticking your tongue in someone's mouth takes practice and communication.

5. If you are happy on your level, stay there for a while. Don't rush; enjoy the scenery. Don't go somewhere just because everyone else is moving on. "Everyone else" may know less than you do. They may be showing off. Americans tend to rush through the sexual levels. The age for first intercourse experience continues to go down, while our collective sexual ignorance goes up.

6. Don't lie about what level you're on just to impress someone. Having intercourse is probably lied about more than taxes.

7. If you are involved in a level of sexual expression but are ashamed to admit it, take that as a signal that you're functioning on the wrong level. If you are lying about how much fun it is, you may have started too soon or gotten incorrect instruction. Go back a level or two if you don't feel comfortable with the level you're on.

Any way you look at it, anything we do at any time in our lives requires certain tools and correct information. If those of us with sexual experience would talk honestly with our peers and younger people, beginners would have a better chance of becoming sexually proud and confident.

We need sexual mentors! Fourteen-year-olds won't know that intercourse is not for beginners unless we share truthful and intimate details about it. We ought to spell out the proper sexual activities for their age. Yes, you can kiss, touch, and rub with your clothes on. It feels good. It works. It's called sex. Enjoy it! Don't move on to the next level without talking to an expert who will give you honest and correct information. Don't forget the emotional and spiritual ramifications, too. They matter just as much. We've pushed through sexual levels too far, too fast, and now we are horrified that the differentiations have all but disappeared. There are no beginners, it seems. If we want each new generation to sexually act their age, then we must do the same. Those of us who are ready must be true sex experts, and we should enjoy being wise teachers and mentors.

19

You Rub Me the Right Way

No one ever talks about one of the best forms of sexual expression: rubbing. I've always appreciated it. I can remember rubbing against furniture as a kid. Now I know about my clitoris. Then, it didn't matter, as long as it felt good. Once I found my four-year-old daughter sliding up and down the kitchen table leg. Like mother, like daughter, I thought. I didn't stop her. I didn't grab the camcorder, either.

When I got to be ten years old, I rubbed with my girlfriend, and we took turns being the boy. We cuddled in bed during sleep-overs and rubbed, one on top of the other. It was fun. It felt good. She was my best friend, and we were in charge. No one was forcing us, and we didn't hurt each other.

A Man to Rub

In high school I met Jimmy, who became my boyfriend. Jimmy and I turned his old clunker of an automobile into a rubber's hideaway on wheels. Early in our relationship we developed a technique of whole body rubbing (WBR). As we kissed, our hands roamed some—a touch on the breast, back, thigh, inner thigh, butt—but soon our hands were needed to hold ourselves in a horizontal position. He was shyer than I was and less assertive, so I ended up on top. We didn't say anything to each other during these mad make-out WBR sessions, but we knew that they were working for both of us. I could feel his erection through my jeans and his. He would have to arrange it so it pointed up to his waist for maximum stimulation. If I lay on top and rubbed my crotch on his erection, we could both have an orgasm. These were quiet, shy orgasms. We knew we were each having one or two, and we knew when they were happening, but we didn't shout "Yahoo." We just opened our eyes and smiled at each other, sweaty and gooey and happy.

In the other cars parked near us on Common Lane, most of my girlfriends were having intercourse. In the locker room the next day, the boys would brag. The girls, however, worried about pregnancy. All that worry and embarrassment, and they weren't even having orgasms.

Mom's Idea

My boyfriend and I had a good thing going. My mom was cool about all this. Actually she gave me the idea to rub instead of having intercourse. First, she gave me all the sex information I wanted, and she gave it honestly, with explicit details. She talked about the emotional aspects as well as the physical.

She knew that we'd go parking on Common Lane. She believed me when I said that we weren't "going all the way." She trusted me, which helped me trust myself. One thing did concern her quite a bit: carbon monoxide poisoning. On cold New England nights she worried that to get some heat, we would keep the car running too long and we'd end up asphyxiated from the fumes. What a mom.

One exceptionally cold night, when police were

known to be hassling parkers, she suggested that we park in front of the house. As reluctant as I was at first to make out with my mom practically watching, I had to admit that her reasoning made sense. Police banging on the car window is a definite orgasm buster. Somehow I convinced Jimmy to go along. After the hockey game we pulled up, shut off the lights and motor, and got horizontal. In the course of an hour, we turned the car on three times for a few minutes each, to warm up a bit.

We're Not Dead, Mom, Okay?

Naturally, those three times were the only three times my mother peeked out the window to make sure we were okay. She panicked! She couldn't see us, and the car had been running for what she thought was over an hour. She dashed out of the house in robe and slippers and flung open the passenger-side door. I looked up behind me from my on-top horizontal position to see my relieved mother closing the door, saying, "It's okay, you're alive, carbon monoxide poisoning, it's okay, go back, sorry . . . carbon monoxide . . . sorry . . . it's okay."

The front door closed behind her, I burst out laughing, and Jimmy looked as if he were going to throw up. I tried to explain my mother's carbon monoxide phobia, but he was convinced that she hated him. I dragged him into the house (any hope of trying to finish lovemaking that night had been lost), and my mom made us some coffee. She elaborated to Jimmy about her fear of carbon monoxide and apologized for embarrassing us. We started talking about sex, as my mom and I did often, and I saw that Jimmy was amazed and totally absorbed. I knew that Jimmy never *ever* talked to his mom or dad about sex. In fact, the only discussion that they'd ever had was when Jimmy was twelve or thirteen years old and stole some condoms from a drugstore. They told him he was a sinner beyond redemption and would suffer in purgatory for thousands of years—if he was lucky. I left Jimmy and my mom sitting at the table, and I went to bed. They talked for hours.

Rubbing Works

This rubbing thing worked for us, and I couldn't understand why all my friends didn't do it instead of intercourse. Probably no one had ever told them that they could. To them, sex meant intercourse. Girls had to fix erections, and boys made the decision on how they wanted their erections fixed. Girls felt responsible for creating these throbbing rods and blue balls.

As women we now know that we don't have to be the designated erection fix-meisters. Everyone can be liberated by rubbing. Tell your friends! Rub me the right way! Rub me 'til I'm raw. Rub me all through the night.

Giving Him the Cold Crotch

I hear a lot of women complain to each other about how they hate some men's lovemaking techniques or lack thereof! Women exchange stories of their breasts getting squeezed like he's trying to get the last drop of shampoo from an empty tube. Or of men rubbing their crotches like Aladdin's lamp, hoping to coax a big-breasted "Genie" out of their vaginas. Hey, it's partly our fault, too. All we have to do is:

1. Stop it before it becomes a bad habit. If you're worried about hurting his feelings or are too shy to say anything, you're not ready to be in that situation. *Go home!*

2. Speak up and instruct your partner. I have found very few men who don't respond favorably to instruction. Most want to know and want to learn. You can do this kindly, with consideration for his feelings.
3. Don't let anyone do anything that you don't like or want. Letting someone do something implies consent on your part.

Suffering in silence and then getting resentful later only makes matters worse. I'd feel angry and confused if all of a sudden, after my partner has gone months or years without saying anything, I'm blasted as a lover, or worse, given the cold shoulder (cold crotch).

    Honest communication shows self-respect as well as respect for your partner and the relationship.

I hear men complain a lot about how unresponsive and unassertive women are during sex, all kinds of sex. Men's laments include: she just lies there; I'm doing all the work; she never comes after me; and, I don't even know if she is getting satisfied!

Well, it's partly men's fault, too!

• If you always make the first move and have for months or years, you have helped to set up the imbalance. Explain how you feel about always being the instigator and admit that you have contributed to the unequal sexual routine. Back off. Take more time and teach and encourage your partner how to be more assertive. Remember: as women, we are less encouraged to be assertive in all areas of life, especially sexuality. Teach us; be our cheerleaders.

- Be careful that once she does make a move, you don't unconsciously take over. I had this experience just recently. I pointed out that whenever we start to kiss, he always has his tongue in my mouth and that it's hard for me to get some control of the kissing activity. He thought about it and agreed to back off a bit and let me start and direct our kissing routine. Also, we agreed that I should also drive the car more often when we travel together!
- Exchange sex roles and play the other person's part so that you get to experience your partner's point of view and positions. I play a great guy, and we get a kick out of how good we can exchange roles. Sometimes, one partner can only get "turned on" by being the aggressor or the passive receiver. Remember that this is a learned response, and instead of unlearning that tried-and-true way to sexual excitement, practice learning additional ways. Just be open in our attitude—that is what really makes positive change possible.

Remember that two people contribute to an imbalance, so it will take two to undo it. And, if one partner is unhappy in the sex life, that means that 50% of the team is not happy or working successfully. No sports team would ever support that kind of imbalance. It's not only a give and take; it's a learn and teach and teach and learn.

20

7here's No Such Thing as a Silly Sex Question

I've been asked everything imaginable. Here are some of the most asked, most embarrassing sex questions—answered! *Questions Women Ask:*

Q. *I know I feel something, but . . . How will I know when I'm having an orgasm?*

A. Think of your vagina throwing up. It's like that but so much more. First of all, the orgasm starts from the clitoris. When pleasurable feelings go out from the clitoris, all your muscles tense up, and the pelvic area, including the vagina, goes into involuntary spasms. Something like vaginal sneezes. A finger inside the vagina while you're having an orgasm will feel the whole vagina contract and squeeze. Juice will flow and your heart will pound. It might make you moan or yell. It might take your breath away. You can have near orgasms, where you approach right to the moment but don't actually go into spasms.

Q. *How long does it take for most women to reach orgasm? I worry I'm taking too long!*

A. It takes the right amount of time! Don't rush it, and if your partner is in a hurry, find someone with more time. First of all, let the tension build and encourage the anticipation, not only between each other but within yourself. For most people, reaching orgasm is like climbing a mountain. You climb, or in this case work up to, a peak, but it's not *the* peak yet. Then you go down into a valley, or in this case rest, lose a little concentration, get self-conscious or whatever holds off the explosion, then you build up to the next peak, getting closer each time. Don't force it, encourage it. Don't get mad or frustrated. Relax your muscles. Don't lose your self-confidence, and don't forget that this is play time, not work time. Orgasm time will vary each day with the ups and downs of stress, physical exhaustion, and your mood. Some orgasms will need more attention and encouragement, and some will need only a thought or light touch. An orgasm is encouraged by mental and emotional stimulation, so start psyching yourself up for one. Tell your partner to slow down, or he can go home and rub himself silly while you relax and enjoy taking your time.

Q. *I can have an orgasm by rubbing and touching myself, but I can't during intercourse.*

A. Good! Women's bodies aren't constructed to have orgasms through intercourse alone. So don't keep trying to have an orgasm relying on his penis. Keep your hand on your clitoris *during* intercourse. If there's no room for your hand, tell him to pull back and give you some room to move. I'm sure this will help you to stimulate yourself and eventually bring you to orgasm.

Q. *Does it hurt the first time you have intercourse?*

A. It can, but it doesn't have to. Most people have intercourse too early. Early in their life, early in their relationship, and early in the night's sexual activity. When a woman is just about to have an orgasm, her vagina is physically ready for intercourse, and as long as there is no medical problem or her partner is not being too rough, there should be no pain.

Q. *Do most women masturbate, and how do they do it? I'm so embarrassed about this, but I really want to know.*

A. This is a hard question to answer, because I'm not convinced that most people tell the truth about their sex lives, specifically their masturbation habits. I know there's all kinds of research about female and male masturbation, and that masturbation is done by both sexes and by most people at some point in their lives. But that's not the real question, or even an important answer. The question is, should we masturbate? How often, and how? Yes, we should, as sexual human beings, masturbate. It's healthy. It teaches us how to please ourselves. It teaches us how to bring ourselves to orgasm, and orgasms are good for us. Orgasms flush out the genital area, lessen headaches, relieve stress, and produce hormones that make us feel happier and more content.

It's fun. It's showing yourself that you like you and that you are worth pleasuring and caressing.

You can, however, masturbate too much. If you are masturbating all day long, all night, not doing your homework, not going to work or spending time with friends. If all you think about and want to do is masturbate, go talk to someone right away. This should not become an obsessive activity. Remember that everyone's sex drive is different, and what might be a lot to one person is not enough for another.

Q. *So, if it's healthy to masturbate, how do I do it?*

A. Touch yourself all over, not just your genitals. Touch your whole body and learn to caress and play. Find out where you like to be touched. Move to your genitals and explore carefully. Don't use anything but your hand at first. Don't use any sharp objects. Don't put anything in your vagina. Some things can be used, but only after you know more about how your genitals work and what can hurt them. Stick with your hands and fingers for now. Use a mirror to see where your clitoris is and how it reacts to pleasure. Vaginal fluid will appear the more you get excited. Use it as a lubricant to help your fingers and hands slide over your genitals. Rubbing is great, and you may be able to rub on something to bring yourself to orgasm. You can put your fingers inside yourself, too. Be careful of fingernails and rings.

So go explore. Find out how you work. Be proud of who you are physically, emotionally, intellectually, spiritually, and sexually.

Q. *I feel so guilty when I make out with a guy and he gets excited. I feel like I have to have intercourse and then I feel worse.*

A. This is such an important comment. You *never* have to have intercourse with someone if you don't want to! Even if you are married. Feeling sorry or feeling obligated is connected to fear and insecurity in sexual situations. Women are brought up to nurture, take care of, and satisfy our man, and to put our needs second to his. Intercourse isn't always used to express love. Don't think that just because he wants to put his penis in your vagina that he loves you. No guy has ever died from blue balls or an unsatisfied erection, and there's no such thing as a tease. Teasing is foreplay, that's the point. A way to avoid this dilemma is to set the record straight at the beginning of making out. "I want to kiss, rub, and touch, but I am not going to have intercourse with you!" Value who *you* are. Don't be a walking semen receptacle.

Questions Men Ask:

Q. *How will I know if my girlfriend is having an orgasm? She gets excited and wet, but I don't know if she's actually coming.*

A. There is one biological manifestation that proves a woman is having an orgasm. The vagina contracts, and you can feel these contractions. If you have your finger inside of her while she's having an orgasm, you will be able to feel the vagina squeeze your finger. And, trust me, women have strong vaginas, so don't expect less than an intense clamp. The other physical manifestations like vaginal fluid, the clitoris filling with blood and becoming hard, heavy breathing and moaning, hard nipples, mean she's getting excited but not necessarily having an orgasm. My advice is to stop having intercourse until you two can show and feel each other's orgasms. Then there's no guessing!

Q. *Most guys I hang out with complain about coming too fast. I'm just the opposite. It takes me a long time to come, and sometimes I just give up. What's wrong?*

A. Are you also embarrassed to pee in front of other guys? Do you try too hard at all you do? Maybe you're too stressed and putting too much pressure on yourself in all areas of your life, including sexually. Guys can have anxiety about their sexuality, too. Slow down! Don't try to have an orgasm. Learn to play and enjoy. Find out how to relax and feel good about yourself without having to perform or reach an orgasm. Get rid of your stress through other outlets like exercise or recreation. And take a look at your emotions. Is anything really bothering you that you're not talking about or that you're denying? All of this can hold off orgasms. By the way, I've never heard a woman complain that her partner took too long.

Q. *I have a hard time holding off my orgasm. I just come too quickly. Is this normal for a young man?*

A. It is, and it also happens to older men. Your sexual response changes throughout your life and is connected to your emotional and physical well-being. Medications can even affect erection and orgasm response. As a young man, it's very common to come quickly. You can practice slowing down by taking a break from your sexual moment. Stop kissing or whatever you're doing and relax for a few minutes. Rub and touch and talk. Don't worry about it; practice helps. If you come, don't panic. Take a breather and keep playing. You'll probably get hard again and maybe even have another orgasm.

Q. *How can I make my girlfriend have an orgasm? She says she doesn't need them, but I feel guilty having all the fun!*

A. Ask her if she wants to know more about herself and her sexuality. She may be harboring guilt or embarrassment from her upbringing or, in some cases, the more serious problem of child abuse. Or she just might not be ready. The problem is that your sex life has become one-way, all for you. No relationship, even friendship or family, should be based on an imbalance of give-and-take. It may be hard, but if I were you, I'd back off and design a sex life you both enjoy. She needs to not feel obligated to satisfy you if she's not getting satisfied herself. On the other hand, having an orgasm is the physically and emotionally healthy result of sexual stimulation. I go back to my original belief that everyone should know how they work before having sex with someone else. I'm sure that she and you enjoy the affection that hopefully is part of your sex together, but it's still not setting a good precedent for either of you. You can't make her have an orgasm, but you can encourage her to explore and masturbate when she's alone and design fun, loving, and mutually satisfying sex when you're together.

So now I'm writing the ending to this book. And my editors pointed out a most important point. I have often used the word "spiritual" in regard to sex, and I guess it's time for me to explain what I mean by that. My spiritual being and energy is my truest and most reliable decision-making voice. I believe we are all inseparable combinations of the physical, emotional, intellectual and spiritual. Most of us let our lives be dictated by only one or two of these aspects, causing an imbalance and repetition of the same good and bad choices and behaviors. How often have I said, "Why do I keep doing that?" Four tools (voices) are better than one or two when fixing a complicated, multi-faceted machine like a human being. Four options (voices) are better than one or two when making important life decisions. Four voices and their distinctive tones are better when combined to sing in harmony. Utilizing the physical, emotional, intellectual and spiritual aspects of our being will create a sex life that contributes to overall successful personal growth.

My spiritual voice, when I encourage it and allow it, is the most thoughtful, reliable, fair and intelligent voice I have. It always comes with concern for me and others. It doesn't always give me the quickest or easiest perspective, but it is always the most truthful. It is the least selfish and most courageous voice I have, but often it is the softest in volume. It can only be as loud as I allow it. It's the least tangible and recognizable, and most difficult to describe. But, I know it's there. It's the easiest to ignore because our world doesn't value it as much as the other three aspects of a person. I have tried sexual experiences without its acknowledged participation, only to discover a nagging uneasy feeling, almost an anxiety, either right after the experience or months later.

Just because we can have a sexual experience devoid of spiritual connection doesn't mean it works or was meant to be that way.

What are the ramifications of building a sex life on one major aspect of your being? From what I've experienced myself and from what others have shared with me, it's a setup for failure—immediately, or down the road.

Physical sex is unfulfilling. The orgasm releases sexual tension, but there's no lasting sensation of having done something worthwhile that can be built upon. It's an experience that often demands re-doing many times to try to reap the most benefits from it. It's a setup. Nothing more than an orgasm can be gained, and its ego boost doesn't last any longer than the orgasm.

Emotional sex often leaves the person feeling more vulnerable. It looks like giving love, but it has its own selfish demands. It's an *I need, I need, I need!*

Intellectual love can be distant, rationalized, polite and devoid of connection. "This is okay to do because we have both agreed that we're smart, sophisticated adults." It's the thinnest sexual experience and is categorized with other analytical decisions based on the facts and information present at the time. It leads and ends nowhere and can't be built upon. It's weak.

Spiritual sex sounds like it should be better, but too many clergy and spiritual leaders have used this same over-spirituality for their own gain, causing pain and trauma to many. It's easy to use the spiritual rationalization to lessen guilt or justify selfish pleasure. People often use spiritual to mean religious. They are not the same. Religion is created by humans; the spiritual is life itself.

The *best* sex life is physical, emotional, intellectual and spiritual. Anything less won't be the best. We deserve the best. Our friends, family and children deserve the best. And the best has no limit and no exclusions. It means *best for all*. Our individual best coming together to make our collective Best Sex Life.

I may have finished this book, but I have not finished trying to build the best sex life, one that is compatible with all my lives and encourages me to create the best family life, work life, play life, community life and love life I can. We can all do it.

TWO VERY PERSONAL THANK-YOUS

To my daughter Kyrsha,

You taught me two of life's most important values. You taught me how to tell the truth and that what I "do" as a mother, woman and person is more important than what I "say." Parents need to thank their children more, because often they give us more than we give back. Thank you for supporting my work, even when it meant sacrifices for you. It is now your turn, and you know I am here and will always be here for you.

I love you, Kyrsha, and could not be more proud of who you are and what you are becoming.

Love always,
Mom

P.S. You can live at home as long as we want!

*   *   *

Dear David,

You are last, but not least!

When I was a little girl and went to a friend's birthday party, the parents always served Neapolitan ice cream. For those of you used to chocolate-chip cookie dough and other "designer" ice cream flavors, the Neapolitan was a rectangular slice of vanilla, strawberry and chocolate ice creams neatly melded together in strips to make a striped canvas cloth motif. I hated it. Here I was looking at my all-time favorite dessert contaminated by two flavors I hated: vanilla and strawberry. So I did what any self-respecting ice cream junkie would do. I ate the strawberry first, because that was my least favorite. I then ate the vanilla, which would help to wash out the strawberry flavor from my mouth, and then I savored the four bites of my all-time favorite flavor, chocolate. I did that with most foods I ate as a kid. Wait, I still do it! I save the best for last. So, here's my best thank-you, and I saved it for last.

You are the chocolate ice cream, and God knows I went through a lot of strawberry and vanilla to get to you. It wasn't that all the strawberry and vanilla were so bad; they just weren't anything like your chocolate. I was afraid for a while that maybe there wasn't a "best" for me. But, with so many people running around this earth, why would I be left without a "best" partner? You were hard to find, but the important thing is that we found each other. I know it sounds clichéd, but it happened when we least expected it and when neither of us was even thinking of looking. I don't believe in coincidence, so it is truly an example of creating reality out of dreams and never giving up on my conviction that we all deserve to love and be loved, gently and honestly.

Best friends and lovers! Thank you for showing me how to put those two together to make a perfect fit, a fit that extends from our minds to our souls, hearts and bodies. Since this book is about changing our sexual attitudes and behaviors, I wouldn't be honest if I didn't thank you for helping me love myself and my sexuality more, to remember to love one another totally (in my four favorite categories— physically, emotionally, intellectually, and spiritually), for loving and teaching Kyrsha what true fatherhood is, for reminding us that it is never too late to have a happy childhood. Your support of Hot, Sexy and Safer through your time and effort is amazing, and you have made me feel more self-worth as a woman and a person than I ever thought possible. I listen and learn from your experience and wisdom and marvel at your commitment to nurturing others.

David, I thank you for being the last and best friend and lover of my life on this earth. I will make a great effort, both in and out of bed, making sure you know how much I appreciate you and am grateful for all you do and all you are. I am proud to be your "buddy."

So now my book is finished. Yet I feel like I just started writing! Maybe because I'm still learning, and ending a book doesn't mean its influence is over. Actually, it's just beginning . . .

All my love and respect,
Suzi

Now that you've read Suzi's book, you're probably dying to see her concert performance of Hot, Sexy and Safer!

To order the Hot, Sexy and Safer concert videotape, send a check made out to Hot, Sexy and Safer for **$15** (includes shipping and handling) to:

>   Hot, Sexy and Safer
>   2461 Santa Monica Blvd., Suite C230
>   Santa Monica, CA 90404

Your name, address and phone number:

_____

_____

_____

phone _____